Injection Techniques in Orthopaedic and Sports Medicine

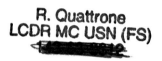

Injection Techniques in Orthopaedic and Sports Medicine

Stephanie Saunders FCSP, FSOM

and

Gordon Cameron MRCGP, FSOM, DMsMED

W. B. SAUNDERS COMPANY LTD
London Philadelphia Toronto Sydney Tokyo

W. B. Saunders Company Ltd

An imprint of Harcourt Brace and Company Limited

First published 1997
Reprinted 1998

A catalogue record for this book is available from the British Library

ISBN 0-7020-2197-0

Phototypeset by J&L Composition, Filey, North Yorkshire
Printed in Great Britain by
Halstan & Company, Amersham, Bucks

CONTENTS

PREFACE

Injection therapy is a useful addition to the treatments employed in combating musculoskeletal pain. It is most effective when combined with rehabilitation regimes such as stretching, strengthening and muscle balancing techniques.

Many patients will obtain lasting symptom relief from a well placed injection, but lack of training, concern about possible side effects and fear of causing the patient more pain make some doctors reluctant to use this approach.

We hope this book will change that. Family practitioners in particular will find it especially useful. It is aimed at a readership of doctors but also of chartered physiotherapists trained in this skill.

Since December 1995 injection therapy officially came within the scope of practice of British chartered physiotherapists, provided they undertake adequate post graduate training. One of us (Stephanie Saunders) has designed and conducts an approved Masters level course to train physiotherapists in the safe and appropriate use of injection therapy.

Along with the Chartered Society of Physiotherapy and the Eli Lilly National Audit Centre we have been establishing national clinical guidelines for injection therapy, particularly in relation to audit and outcome. Both authors conduct courses in Orthopaedic Medicine internationally and further information about these courses and clinical guidelines can be obtained from the address below.

In order to make the book easy to use we have simplified each technique and present only the essential facts. Giving injections is easy; selection of the appropriate patient is difficult. The *main points* in the history and examination are given to aid the reader in this selection.

While we suggest the use of triamcinolone acetonide throughout the book as it appears to cause less afterpain, any appropriate corticosteroid may be used.

We owe special thanks to Dr James Cyriax for his pioneering work in the use of injectable corticosteroids, to Dr Richard Ellis and Dr Stephen Longworth for their useful advice, and to Lynne Gardner for her uncomplaining and tireless work in helping to bring this book to fruition.

Stephanie Saunders MCSP   Gordon Cameron MB BS

Orthopaedic Medicine Seminars
20 Ailsa Road
Twickenham
TW1 1QW
ENGLAND

CORTICOSTEROIDS

Steroid drugs have had a bad press in recent years. Many members of the public are worried about them and this fear is sometimes shared by those in the medical and paramedical professions. But if steroid drugs are used properly the potential benefits vastly outweigh their side effects.

The art of good injection therapy is to place an appropriate amount of an appropriate drug into the affected tissue.

Problems with steroid use arise when:

- too large a dose is used,

- an inappropriate drug is chosen,

- injections are given too frequently and

- poor injection technique allows spread of the drug to adjacent tissues.

HOW DO STEROIDS WORK?

Steroid drugs act in two ways within the body:

as *glucocorticoids* – suppressers of the inflammatory response

or

as *mineralocorticoids* – modifiers of salt and water balance.

Different steroid agents have the above properties in different proportions and Table 1 illustrates how they compare.

Only those with a large anti-inflammatory (glucocorticoid) and low fluid balance effect (mineralocorticoid) are useful in treating musculoskeletal problems.

Triamcinolone and prednisolone are best suited for use in the injection techniques we describe in this book. Hydrocortisone acetate may sometimes be used – it has a shorter duration of action in the tissues and is more soluble.

Steroids also differ in the potency of their anti-inflammatory effect and in the duration of their action within the tissues (Table 2).

Most people using steroid injections in musculoskeletal disorders use triamcinolone or methylprednisolone. We prefer triamcinolone — the available preparations offer more flexibility in dosage and the drug is more soluble in local anaesthetic solutions. In our experience it also seems to give less pain after injection than the other drugs.

Table 1   Properties of steroid drugs

DRUG	GLUCOCORTICOID (ANTI-INFLAMMATORY) EFFECT	MINERALOCORTICOID (FLUID BALANCE EFFECT)
FLUDROCORTISONE	+	+++++
CORTISONE	++	+++
HYDROCORTISONE	+++	++
PREDNISOLONE	++++	+
METHYL PREDNISOLONE	++++	+
TRIAMCINOLONE	++++	+
BECLOMETHASONE	++++	+

Table 2   Common steroid preparations

DRUG	DOSE	POTENCY	MANUFACTURER
SHORT ACTING	25 mg/ml	+	
HYDROCORTISONE ACETATE	1 ml		KNOLL PHARMA
(HYDROCORTISTAB)	AMPOULES		
INTERMEDIATE ACTING	40 mg/ml	+++++	
METHYLPREDNISOLONE	1 ml, 2 ml, 3 ml		UPJOHN
(DEPO-MEDRONE)	VIALS		
TRIAMCINOLONE ACETONIDE	10 mg/ml		SQUIBB
(ADCORTYL)	1 ml AMPOULES 5 ml VIALS		
(KENALOG)	40 mg/ml 1 ml VIALS		SQUIBB
TRIAMCINOLONE HEXACETONIDE (LEDERSPAN)	20 mg/ml 1 ml OR 5 ml VIALS		LEDERLE
LONG-ACTING		+++++++	
DEXAMETHASONE	4 mg/ml	+++++++	M.S.D
(DECADRON)	2 ml VIALS		

Table 3   Side effects of steroid injection

SYSTEMIC SIDE EFFECTS	LOCAL SIDE EFFECTS
FLUSHING OF THE SKIN	INFECTION
MENSTRUAL IRREGULARITY	SUBCUTANEOUS ATROPHY
MUSCLE WASTING AND MYOPATHY	SKIN DEPIGMENTATION
IMPAIRED GLUCOSE TOLERANCE	TENDON RUPTURE
OSTEOPOROSIS	
PSYCHOLOGICAL UPSET	
STEROID ARTHROPATHY	
ADRENAL SUPPRESSION	

INDICATIONS FOR CORTICOSTEROID INJECTION

Steroids are indicated whenever the lesion being treated has an inflammatory component. Chapter 5, which deals with the individual conditions, gives details of dosage, volume of injection and suggested frequency of treatment.

SIDE EFFECTS OF STEROID INJECTION

Systemic effects

All drugs given by injection have both a local and a systemic effect. The larger the dose, the greater the systemic effect.

Two systemic effects are frequently seen, the others are rare.

Flushing – commonly when doses of greater than 20 mg of triamcinolone (or equivalent) are given.

Menstrual irregularity – occurs when women are given doses higher than 40 mg triamcinolone.

Rare but recognized other side effects are:

Impaired glucose tolerance – warn diabetics that this may occur. It is transient.

Osteoporosis – only seen when high doses are given over long periods of time.

Table 4   Avoidable local side effects

SIDE EFFECT	CAUSE
SKIN DAMAGE ATROPHY DEPIGMENTATION DISCOLORATION	POOR TECHNIQUE I.E. TOO LARGE A DOSE TOO MUCH VOLUME TOO OFTEN A DOSE SUBCUTANEOUS INJECTION
TENDON RUPTURE	POOR TECHNIQUE I.E. TOO LARGE A VOLUME TOO MUCH STEROID TOO OFTEN INJECTED BOLUS INJECTION

Psychological disturbance – euphoria or paranoia; high doses may induce aggression.

Steroid arthropathy – probably only occurs with the use of oral steroids for serious medical illness. Injection of steroids into joints has never been convincingly shown to cause arthropathy unless grossly excessive doses are given repeatedly over a long period of time. Rheumatoid joints are particularly at risk:

Muscle wasting and myopathy – really only seen with long-term oral steroid use.

Immunosuppression – resistance to infection is diminished in *all* patients who have been injected with steroid. The effect is transient but the bigger the dose of steroid, the more prolonged the effect. Viral infections such as chickenpox may be particularly dangerous.

A note on steroid cards

The government has produced a card to be carried by the patient and intended to warn of the dangers of steroid therapy. It is designed for those taking long-term oral therapy and the warnings it carries do not apply to one-off injections of steroid.

It is not our practice to issue one of these cards to patients treated by injection for a musculoskeletal problem. We do however always spend time explaining the above issues and giving simple instruction on what the patient can expect in the following days and weeks.

Local side effects

The local side effects of steroid injection are common. Some, such as post-injection flare are unavoidable and transient. Most of the others are the result of poor technique (Table 4).

Post injection flare – is probably due to the transient precipitation of small crystals within the tissue fluids. The patient experiences a temporary worsening of their pain and sometimes swelling and local heat. It can be difficult to differentiate this from septic arthritis but the latter is much rarer and usually associated with fever and an ill patient. The flare reaction will settle quickly if an oral NSAID (non-steroidal anti-inflammatory drug) is given. Some steroid preparations seem more prone to producing a flare reaction than others; we seldom find problems when using triamcinolone.

There are three main uses for local anaesthetic drugs in orthopaedic medical practice:

- *as an aid to diagnosis;*
- *to diminsh pain;*
- *to provide volume to injections of steroid.*

An aid to diagnosis

Even the most experienced practitioner will sometimes be unsure exactly which tissue is at fault. Make a best guess at the tissue at fault; inject a small amount of local anaesthetic into only that tissue; wait a few moments and then re-examine. If the pain is relieved then the 'guilty party' has been identified and treatment can be accurately directed.

Pain relief

If the guidelines we give for injection techniques are followed then most patients will find the procedures relatively painless. We do not routinely use skin anaesthesia prior to injections. We do, however, recommend mixing a steroid drug and local anaesthetic in the same syringe and injecting both simultaneously. This allows temporary relief of pain in the target tissue while the steroid begins its anti-inflammatory action. The effect of the local also allows immediate retesting of function as a check that the drug has reached its intended destination.

Mixing steroids with local anaesthetics

Although one proprietary brand of steroid is available ready mixed with local anaesthetic we don't find this useful in clinical practice. The dose and volume are fixed at 40 mg steroid per millilitre and this does not allow for flexibility of dosage. We also think that using this product often tempts the practitioner to inject a larger dose of steroid than is appropriate for the tissue being treated. It is much better simply to mix the two drugs to your own requirements. This allows an almost limitless combination of doses and volumes.

   Some steroid drugs mix better with local anaesthetics than others. Hydrocortisone acetate is very soluble and forms an almost clear solution when mixed. Methylprednisolone is the opposite – it forms a visible crystal sediment in the syringe. The triamcinolone preparations lie between these two extremes and form a non-crystalline milky solution.

AVAILABLE LOCAL ANAESTHETIC PREPARATIONS

Table 5 outlines the differences between commonly used local anaesthetics.

Table 5   Local anaesthetics: time to onset and duration of action

DRUG	TIME FROM INJECTION TO ONSET OF EFFECT (MIN)	DURATION OF ACTION
LIGNOCAINE	1–2	~1 h
PRILOCAINE	1–2	~1 h
PROCAINE	1	30 min
BUPIVACAINE	≤ 30	≤ 8 h

HOW DO LOCAL ANAESTHETICS WORK?

All local anaesthetics in use today have the same basic chemical structure as cocaine. The differences between them lie in the side chains of molecules attached to the basic chemical structure.

They all act by causing a reversible block to impulse conduction along nerve fibres.

The smallest fibres are most easily blocked, so that the blocking of pain and other nerve functions is dose-related (Fig.1).

This type of differential block is only relevant when large doses of local anaesthetic are used. The volumes and doses recommended in this book should produce only relief of pain and loss of skin sensation.

EFFECTS OF LOCAL ANAESTHETICS

All local anaesthetic drugs have both local and systemic effects.

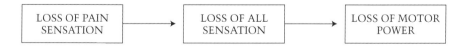

| LOSS OF PAIN SENSATION | → | LOSS OF ALL SENSATION | → | LOSS OF MOTOR POWER |

AS DOSE OF LOCAL ANAESTHETIC INCREASES

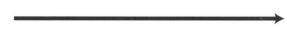

Fig 1

The duration of the local effect depends upon how quickly the drug is taken away from the local site by the bloodstream. This in turn depends on the specific drug and also on the amount of blood supply to the area injected.

It can be dangerous to inject a large volume of local anaesthetic into a very inflamed (and thus very vascular) part of the body as very rapid uptake will occur and systemic effects may be seen.

Sometimes local anaesthetics are mixed with adrenaline to deliberately slow down the rate of systemic absorption. This is neither recommended nor necessary for the techniques discussed in this book.

TOXIC SIDE EFFECTS OF LOCAL ANAESTHETICS

Side effects due to overdosage

Both the heart and the brain may be adversely affected. The early signs are excitation of the nervous system. The patient may feel drunk and experience tingling around the lips and tongue. A sensation of agitation or anxiety may be experienced and this can progress to convulsions, coma and respiratory arrest.

Table 6 shows the volume of local anaesthetic above which side effects may be expected. Do note that side effects are in part dependent on the patients reaction to the drug and can occur with doses lower than the maximum. The doses listed are for a healthy adult of medium build.

Table 6   Doses of local anaesthetic above which systematic toxicity is likely

DRUG		MAXIMAL VOLUME
LIGNOCAINE	0.5%	40 ml
	1.0%	20 ml
(XYLOCAINE)	2.0%	10 ml
BUPIVACAINE	0.25%	60 ml
	0.5 %	30 ml
(MARCAINE)		
PRILOCAINE	0.5%	80 ml
	1.0%	40 ml
(CITANEST)	2.0%	20 ml
PROCAINE	0.5%	200 ml
	1.0%	100 ml
	2.0%	50 ml

N.B. These volumes refer to the use of the plain drug without the addition of adrenaline.

Side effects due to allergy

Always ask about previous allergic problems before giving an injection of local anaesthetic. Allergic reactions may be mild, delayed and of nuisance value only or they may be catastrophic, immediate and potentially fatal.

All those using local anaesthetic injections should have the rescucitation facilities to cope with cardiac or respiratory arrest due to unexpected severe allergic reactions.

The warning signs are flushing, itching and the appearance of urticaria. The patient may feel chest tightness, abdominal pain or nausea. They can become wheezy or vomit. Total circulatory collapse and death may follow. **These warning signs may be totally absent** and the patient may collapse without warning anytime up to 30 minutes after the injection.

SAFETY PROCEDURES

ASEPTIC TECHNIQUE

- Use only pre-packed sterile disposable needles and syringes.

- Use single dose ampoules where possible

- Change needles after drawing up your solution into the syringe.

- Use domestically clean and dry hands – wet hands carry a greater risk of infection

- Neither scrubbing up nor gowning is required. Gloves are not normally necessary but in some countries are mandatory.

- Mark the skin site with a retracted ballpen or your finger nail and cleanse with alcohol or an izodine-based solution. Do not touch the skin thereafter.

- Do not guide the needle with your finger.

- When injecting a joint, aspirate first to ensure that you are in the joint space and check that the fluid does not look infected. If in doubt do not inject steroid and send the joint fluid for bateriological analysis.

ANTICIPATION OF PROBLEMS

Problems are rare but be prepared for them in advance.
The two most common are:

- fainting;
- severe allergic reactions.

Fainting

The usual causes of a faint during injection are *pain, apprehension or needle phobia*.
The patient will usually get a warning of the impending faint but this is not always the case.

Treatment

- *Lie the patient supine and elevate the legs;*
- *reassure them strongly that they will shortly recover;*
- *if they lose consciousness briefly, then protect the airway and give oxygen at 35% concentration.*

Problems with patients who faint only arise when the patient is kept upright, when convulsions may occur due to cerebral hypoxia.

If your patient is anxious then the first injection is best given in a lying position. Beware the stoic who insists on having the injection in the upright position, they often faint when least expected.

Severe allergic reactions

Some patients are allergic to local anaesthetic preparations. They may not be aware of this. A previous uneventful injection is not a guarantee that they will not be allergic this time, although it does provide a degree of reassurance.

If a reaction occurs it is usually seen immediately but can be delayed for up to 30 minutes. If in any doubt do not let your patient leave your clinic until you are sure they have recovered.

Early warning signs of allergy

- *Flushing,*
- *itching,*
- *urticaria.*

These early signs may be entirely absent

Signs of severe allergy are

- *Wheezing,*
- *chest tightness,*
- *abdominal pain,*
- *nausea and vomiting.*

Circulatory collapse, cardiac arrest and death may follow.

The treatment of severe allergic reactions

- *Establish intravenous access immediately,*
- *maintain an airway,*
- *seek help.*

Give

- Oxygen – 35% by mask.

- Adrenaline 1:1000 – 1 ml intramuscularly or subcutaneously to combat shock and circulatory collapse.

- Dipheniramine (piriton) – 20 mg intravenously to counteract the excessive histamine release.

- Hydrocortisone – 200 mg intravenously to suppress any further allergic reaction.

Arrange admission to hospital for observation.

EMERGENCY SUPPLIES FOR THE TREATMENT ROOM

All those using drugs by injection should have a supply of emergency equipment and medication at hand. Problems are rare but do happen. Having the emergency kit available does not guarantee a successful outcome but failure to have it would be legally indefensible.

Suggested emergency kit

- A supply of disposable plastic airways;

- a selection of IV canulae and fluid-giving sets;

- normal saline for infusion;

- plasma substitute for infusion;

- oxygen with masks and tubing;

- an ambubag and mask for assisted ventilation;

- needles and syringes for injection;

- adrenaline 1:1000 strength.

- piriton 20 mg for injection.

- hydrocortisone for injection.

All drugs and fluids should be checked regularly to ensure they do not go out of date.

GUIDELINES TO USING THE INJECTION TECHNIQUES

The fifth chapter illustrates the injection techniques used most often in clinical practice for lesions of the upper and lower limb.

In order to simplify the instructions and enable the practitioner to follow them easily, information is kept to a minimum. The following guidelines should therefore be studied carefully before using any of the techniques.

Headings

Each page covers one anatomical structure with the most common lesion found there.

Causes and findings

Giving injections is easy; the difficult part is diagnosis and selection of suitable treatment. Great care must be taken in objective and subjective assessment with a clear knowledge of the indications and contraindications of the therapy. To aid in selection of appropriate patients, the common causes of the lesion and the main findings of the assessment are listed.

Equipment

The instruction tables show the recommended size of syringe and needle, dosage and volume of corticosteroid and local anaesthetic. These doses and volumes are usual for the average adult, but may be adapted for smaller or larger frames. Always consider the strength and the volume required and choose needle and syringe of a size appropriate for the structure and volume to be injected. All needles and syringes must be of single-use disposable type.

Syringes

Have available 1 ml, 2 ml, 5 ml, 10 ml and 20 ml syringes. Rarely a 50 ml syringe is necessary.

Use a small bore 1 ml tuberculin syringe for small tendons and ligaments as the resistance of the structure requires a considerable amount of pressure. Considerable back pressure may cause a larger syringe to blow off the needle and the clinician to be sprayed with the solution – an embarrassing situation.

Needles

Select the finest needle of the appropriate length to reach the lesion. Even on a slim person, it is necessary to use a 2.5 or 3 inch needle to successfully infiltrate deep structures such as the hip joint or psoas bursa. When injecting with a long fine spinal needle, it is useful to keep the trochar in place to help control the needle as it passes through tissue planes.

The following needle sizes and colours are most commonly used and are universally available in Britain. Other countries may use different hub colours.

25 Gauge	(0.5 mm)	Orange	0.5 to 5/8 inch	(13–20 mm)
23 Gauge	(0.6 mm)	Blue	1 to 1.25 inch	(25–30 mm)
21 Gauge	(0.8 mm)	Green	1.5 to 2 inch	(40–50 mm)
19 Gauge	(1.1 mm)	White	1.5 inch	(40 mm)
Spinal 21 or 22 Gauge	(0.7–0.8 mm)	Black	3 inch	(75 mm)

Corticosteroid

Kenalog (Triamcinolone acetonide with 40 mg steroid per ml) is the steroid we usually inject. In our experience it gives less afterpain in tendinous injections than Depomedrone (methyl prednisolone) and is equally effective. Preliminary results of a comparative study support this.

Another advantage is that Kenalog can be used in both small and large areas, although where the total volume to be injected is large the weaker solution, Adcortyl (triamcinolone acetonide with 10 mg steroid per ml), can be used.

Local anaesthetic

Any suitable anaesthetic can be used. We suggest *Xylocaine* 2% in small areas, 1% in larger areas and 0.5% in large areas where more volume is required. Occasionally *Marcain* is used where a longer anaesthetic effect is needed. Some practitioners like to mix a short- and long-acting anaesthetic.

Dosage and volume

The doses and volumes given in the following tables are intended as guidelines only. They are governed by the size and age of the patient, the number of injections to be given and by clinical judgement.

Tendons and ligaments should have the minimum possible amount of volume and steroid inserted. A small volume avoids painful distension of the structure and the small dose minimises risk of rupture. An average 'recipe' for most tendon lesions is 10 mg of steroid in 1 ml of local anaesthetic. Larger structures may require up to 20 mg steroid in 2 ml volume.

Joints and bursae appear to respond best when sufficient fluid to slightly inflate the capsule or bursa is introduced. Possibly the slight distension 'splints' the structure or, perhaps, breaks down some adhesions.

Recommended maximum dosages and volumes in joint injections for an average-sized person are shown in Tables 7 and 8. In a small patient the amounts are decreased. These volumes are well within safety limits and will not cause the capsule to rupture, for instance it is not unusual to aspirate 80 ml of blood from an injured knee joint. In any case, the back pressure created by too large a volume would blow the syringe off the fine needle recommended well before the capsule was compromised.

Table 7   Approximate maximum volumes for joint injections

SHOULDER	10 ml	HIP	5 ml
ELBOW	5 ml	KNEE	10 ml
WRIST	2 ml	ANKLE	3 ml
THUMB, FINGERS	1 ml	TOES	1.5 ml

Table 8   Approximate maximum dosages for joint injections

SHOULDER	30 mg	HIP	40 mg
ELBOW	20 mg	KNEE	40 mg
WRIST, THUMB	10 mg	ANKLE, FOOT	20 mg
FINGERS	5 mg	TOES	10 mg

Anatomy

As an aid to identifying the structures, we have given tips for simple ways to remember individual sizes and to localise them based on functional and surface anatomy. Where finger sizes are given, the refer to the *patient's* fingers, not the examiner's.

Technique

Injections should *not* be painful. Skin is very sensitive, especially on the flexor surfaces of the body, and bone is equally so. Muscles, tendons and ligaments are less sensitive and cartilage virtually insensitive. Pain caused at the time of the injection is invariably the result of poor technique – *hitting* bone with the needle instead of *caressing* it. Afterpain can be caused by a traumatic periostitis because of damaging bone with the needle, or possibly by 'flare' caused by the type of steroid used. Success does not depend on a painful flare after the infiltration, although some patients do
experience this. It is good practice to warn patients of possible afterpain and to ensure that they have painkillers available should they need them.

The secret of giving a reasonably comfortable treatment depends on using the needle as an extension of the finger. The needle should be inserted quickly perpendicular to the skin and then passed gently through the tissue planes, feeding back information about the structures from the consistency of those tissues. The usual 'feel' of different tissues is as follows:

- *Muscle – spongy, soft*

- *Tendon or ligament – fibrous, tough*

- *Capsule – often slight resistance to the needle, like pushing through rubber top of ampoule*

- *Cartilage – sticky, toffee-like*

- *Bone – hard*

Bursae and joint capsules

These are hollow structures requiring a *bolus technique*. No resistance to the introduction of fluid indicates that the needle tip is intra-capsular or within the bursa. Chronic bursitis often results in loculation of the bursa; this gives the sensation of pockets of free flow and resistance within the bursa, rather like injecting a sponge.

Tendons and ligaments

These require a *peppering technique*. This helps to disperse the solution through-out the structure and to eliminate the possibility of rupture. The needle is gently inserted to caress the bone and the solution is then introduced in little droplets as if into all the areas of a sugar cube. Knowledge of the size of the structure being infiltrated is essential as this decides the volume of fluid required and how much the needle tip has to be moved around. There is only one skin puncture; this is not multiple acupuncture.

Tendons with sheaths: After inserting the needle perpendicular to the skin, the needle is laid alongside the tendon within the sheath and the fluid introduced. Often a small bulge is observed contained within the sheath.

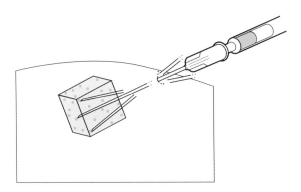

PREPARATION

Discuss the various treatment options, the injection procedure and possible side effects with the patient and obtain their informed consent.

Prepare the following equipment

- Syringe and needles for drawing up and infiltrating
- Spare syringe and sterile container in case aspiration is necessary
- Corticosteroid and local anaesthetic – check drug name, dose and expiry date
- Alcohol swab, industrial methylated spirit, iodine or other suitable skin preparation
- Cotton wool and skin plaster

THE PROCEDURE

- *Patient*

  Place in comfortable sitting or lying position with site accessible.

- *Identify structure*

  Put skin under traction and mark site firmly with finger nail or retracted end of ballpoint pen.

- *Aseptic technique*

  Wash hands with suitable cleanser and dry well with disposable towel. (Most clinicians in Britain do not use sterile gloves unless sepsis is suspected, but in some areas it is mandatory (Haslock et al)).

  Clean skin and allow to dry.

  Clean rubber bungs and open vials.

  Draw up steroid first and then local anaesthetic to required volume.

  Attach a fresh needle of correct size firmly to the syringe.

- *Insert needle*

  Use no touch sterile technique.

  Draw back on plunger to make sure tip is not in artery or vein.

  Avoid puncturing large blood vessel — if this occurs, apply firm pressure over site for 5 (vein) or 10 minutes (artery).

  Avoid injecting large volumes of air — small air bubbles are no problem unless intravascular.

  Check any aspirated fluid — if sepsis suspected, aspirate with fresh syringe and deposit in sterile container for culture. Abandon injection.

- *Introduce solution*

  Use bolus technique for joints or bursae.

  Use peppering technique for tendons and ligaments.

  Never inject into body of achilles or infrapatellar tendons.

- *Withdraw needle*

  Press on site with cotton wool.

  Dispose of needle and syringe immediately into 'sharps' container.

  Apply plaster if necessary – check for allergy to this first.

- *Record*

  Drug names, doses and batch numbers.

  Aseptic technique.

  Advice and warnings about response to injection.

- *Reassess patient*

  Record result of treatment on pain, power and range.

17

Aftercare

The ideal outcome is total relief of pain with normal power and range of motion. This does not always occur but there should be significant immediate improvement to encourage both patient and clinician that the correct diagnosis has been made and the injection accurately placed.

Explain the probable after effects of the injection to the patient. The relief of pain will be temporary, depending on the strength and type of anaesthetic used, and the pain may return when the effect of the anaesthetic wears off. Some patients describe this pain to be more than their original pain, but this is usually short lived. This may be due to the flare effect which is thought to be caused by microcrystal deposition. It may also be that pain which comes back after a break may *appear* to be worse.

Any afterpain can be eased by application of ice or taking non-steroidal anti-inflammatory medication or simple analgesics.

The anti-inflammatory effect of the corticosteroid is not usually apparent until 36 to 48 hours after the infiltration and may continue for up to three weeks depending on the drug used.

Arrange to review the patient about a week or ten days later, or sooner if the pain is severe or begins to return; as in acute capsulitis of the shoulder.

Relative rest means that the normal activities of daily living can be followed providing they are not painful. The patient should be encouraged to continue to do anything that is comfortable. If the symptoms were caused by overuse, the sport or repetitive activity should not be engaged upon until the patient has been passed as fit.

Once the symptoms have been relieved, the patient must be advised on rehabilitation and prevention of recurrence. This may involve adaptation of movement patterns, correction of posture, stretching and or strengthening regimes. The advice of a professional coach or expert in orthotics may also be required.

Comments

In this section we have listed the expected results of the treatment, complications that may occur and appropriate alternative approaches to treating the lesion described.

INJECTION TECHNIQUES

Acute or chronic capsulitis — 'frozen shoulder'

Cause

Trauma.

Osteoarthritis or rheumatoid arthritis.

Idiopathic.

Findings

Pain in deltoid area possibly radiating down to hand.

Painful loss of: *most* passive lateral rotation with a hard end feel;

less passive abduction;

least passive medial rotation.

Equipment

SYRINGE	NEEDLE	KENALOG 40	LOCAL ANAESTHETIC
10 ml	21G 1.5" – 2" (0.8 × 40–50 mm)	30 mg	8–10 ml 0.5%

Anatomy

The shoulder joint is surrounded by a large capsule and the easiest and least painful approach is posteriorly. There are no major blood vessel or nerves lying here. An imaginary oblique line running from the posterior angle of the acromion to the coracoid process anteriorly passes through the shoulder joint. The needle follows this line, passing through deltoid, infraspinatus and posterior capsule.

Technique

- *Patient sits with arm held in medial rotation across waist.*
- *Identify posterior angle of acromion with thumb and coracoid process anterior with index finger.*
- *Insert needle just below angle and push obliquely anterior towards coracoid process. End point is when needle touches intra-articular cartilage.*
- *Introduce fluid in a bolus.*

Aftercare

Maintenance of mobility within the pain free range with stronger stretching when pain free.

Comments

The less the radiation of pain and the earlier the joint is treated, the more dramatic is the relief of symptoms. Usually one injection is successful in the early stages of the condition, but if necessary more can safely be given at increasing intervals of 1 week, 10 days, etc. Rarely the posterior approach is not effective so then an anterior approach can be used. In this case, the arm is held in lateral rotation and the needle is inserted anteriorly between the coracoid process and the lesser tuberosity of the humerus and aimed posteriorly towards the spine of the scapular. The same volume and dose is used.

20

SHOULDER JOINT

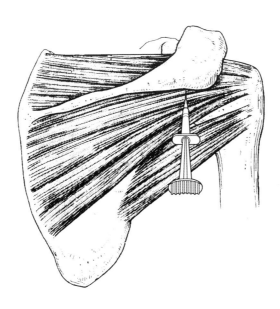

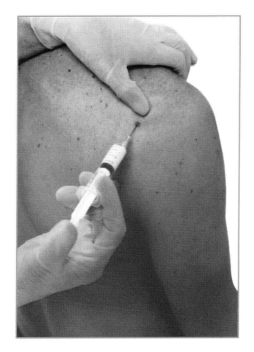

Acute or chronic capsulitis

Cause

Trauma.
Occasionally prolonged overuse.

Findings

Pain at point of shoulder.

Pain at extreme of range of all passive movements, especially full passive horizontal adduction.

Occasional painful arc.

Equipment

SYRINGE	NEEDLE	KENALOG 40	LOCAL ANAESTHETIC
1 ml	25G 0.5" (0.33 × 13 mm)	10 mg	1 ml 2%

Anatomy

The acromio-clavicular joint line runs in the sagittal plane about a thumb's width medial to the edge of the acromion. The joint plane runs obliquely medially and may contain a small meniscus. Often a small step can be palpated where the acromion abuts against the clavicle, or a small V-shaped gap felt at the anterior joint margin.

Technique

- *Patient sits supported with arm hanging by side to slightly separate the joint surfaces.*

- *Identify top of acromion. Move medially about a thumb's width and palpate joint line.*

- *Insert needle angling medially about 30° and pass through capsule.*

- *Deposit solution in a bolus.*

Aftercare

Relative rest for one week then gentle mobilizing exercises.
Acutely inflamed joints are helped by the application of ice and taping to stabilize the joint.

Comments

Occasionally the joint is difficult to enter. Traction on the arm and peppering of the capsule with the solution while feeling for the joint space is recommended.

ACROMIO-CLAVICULAR JOINT

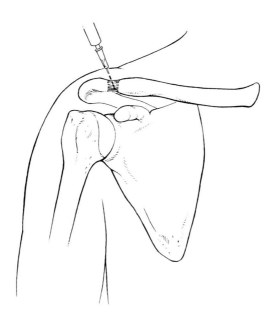

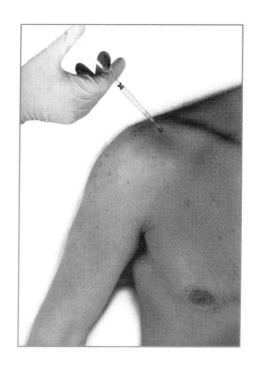

STERNO-CLAVICULAR JOINT

Acute or chronic capsulitis

Causes

Trauma or overuse.

Findings

Pain over sterno-clavicular joint.
Painful: retraction and protraction of the shoulder;
full elevation of the arm;
clicking.

Equipment

SYRINGE	NEEDLE	KENALOG 40	LOCAL ANAESTHETIC
1 ml	25G 0.5" (0.33 × 13 mm)	10 mg	0.75 ml

Anatomy

The sterno-clavicular joint contains a small meniscus which can sometimes give painful symptoms. The joint line runs obliquely laterally from superior to inferior and can be identified by palpating the joint medial to the end of the clavicle while the patient protracts and retracts the shoulder.

Technique

- *Patient lies with arm in lateral rotation.*
- *Identify joint line.*
- *Insert needle perpendicular through joint capsule.*
- *Deposit solution in bolus.*

Aftercare

Rest for a week followed by progressive exercise regime.

Comments

Although not a common lesion, this responds well to one infiltration.

STERNO-CLAVICULAR JOINT

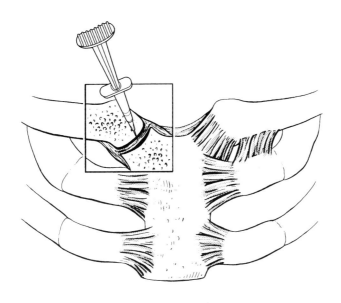

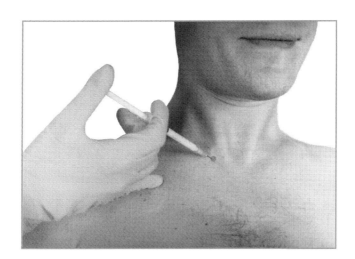

SUPRASPINATUS TENDON

Chronic tendonitis

Cause

Overuse.

Findings

Pain in deltoid area.
Painful: resisted abduction;
         arc on active abduction.

Equipment

SYRINGE	NEEDLE	KENALOG 40	LOCAL ANAESTHETIC
1 ml	25G 1" (0.5 × 25 mm)	10 mg	0.75 ml 2%

Anatomy

The greater tuberosity of the humerus, into which the tendon inserts, lies in direct line with the lateral epicondyle of the elbow. Therefore, palpation of the epicondyle first helps to identify the greater tuberosity, especially on a muscular or fat patient. The tendon is approximately the width of the middle fingertip at the teno-osseous insertion into the superior facet on the tuberosity.

Technique

- *Patient sits supported with forearm medially rotated behind back. This brings the tendon out from under the acromion and into the sagittal plane.*
- *Identify lateral epicondyle of the elbow, now facing anteriorly, and run finger up the front of humerus to anterior edge of the acromion. The greater tuberosity now lies immediately anterior with the tendon in the hollow between the two bones.*
- *Insert needle perpendicular through tendon to touch bone.*
- *Pepper solution into tendon.*

Aftercare

Relative rest for one week then progressive exercise regime and postural control when symptom free.

Comments

Supraspinatus tendonitis can occur on its own but is more commonly associated with subdeltoid bursitis. Always treat the bursa first and if some pain remains on resisted abduction, then the tendon can be infiltrated a week or so later. When the lesion occurs at the musculo-tendinous junction there is no painful arc. Infiltration may not be as successful here and electrotherapy with deep friction can be more effective.

Calcification can arise within the tendon where a hard resistance is felt with the needle. The symptoms often recur but it is worth attempting to break up the calcification with a large bore needle and local anaesthetic. The results are variable. If symptoms persist a surgical opinion should be sought.

26

SUPRASPINATUS TENDON

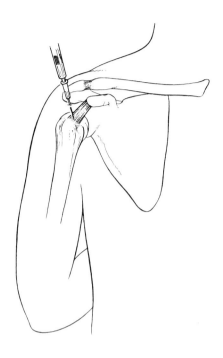

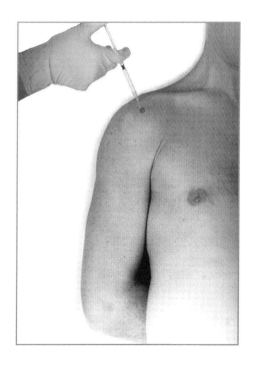

INFRASPINATUS TENDON

Chronic tendonitis

Cause

Overuse.

Findings

Pain in deltoid area.
Painful: resisted lateral rotation;
         arc on active abduction.

Equipment

SYRINGE	NEEDLE	KENALOG 40	LOCAL ANAESTHETIC
2 ml	23G 1.25" (0.6 × 30 mm)	15–20 mg	1.5 ml 1%

Anatomy

The infraspinatus and teres minor tendons insert together into the middle and lower facets on the posterior aspect of the greater tuberosity of the humerus. They are together approximately three fingers wide at the teno-osseous insertion.

Technique

- *Patient sits with supported arm flexed to right angle and held in adduction and lateral rotation. This brings the posterior facets out from under the thickest portion of the deltoid and puts the tendon under tension running obliquely upwards and laterally.*

- *Identify posterior angle of acromion. Tendon insertion now lies 45° inferior and lateral in direct line with lateral epicondyle of elbow.*

- *Insert needle at mid point of tendons at insertion into bone. Pass through deltoid and tendon and touch bone.*

- *Pepper solution in two rows up and down into teno-osseous junction.*

Aftercare

Relative rest for one week then progressive exercise regime and postural correction when symptom free.

Usually a painful arc is present which indicates that the lesion lies at the teno-osseous junction. Occasionally there is no arc when the lesion lies in the body of the tendon. In this case the needle is inserted more medially where there is often an area of tenderness, and the same technique applied.

Comments

The smaller patient is given the smaller amount of volume but for a large man, a greater volume and dose is required.

INFRASPINATUS TENDON

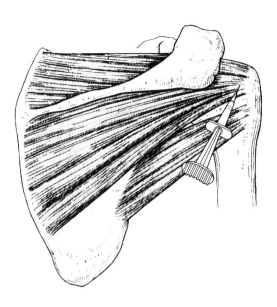

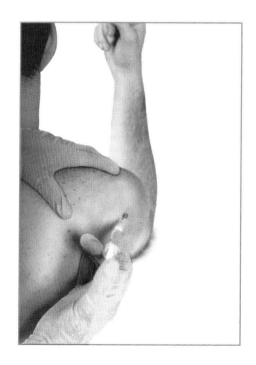

SUBSCAPULARIS TENDON AND BURSA

Acute or chronic tendonitis or bursitis

Cause

Overuse or trauma.

Findings

Pain in deltoid area or anterior to shoulder.
Painful: resisted medial rotation;
      arc on active abduction;
      passive lateral rotation and full passive horizontal adduction (scarf test).

Equipment

SYRINGE	NEEDLE	KENALOG 40	LOCAL ANAESTHETIC
TENDON 1 ml BURSA 2 ml	23G 1.25" (0.6 × 30 mm)	TENDON 10 mg BURSA 20 mg	TENDON 0.75 ml 2% BURSA 2 ml 1%

Anatomy

The subscapularis tendon inserts into the medial edge of the lesser tuberosity of the humerus. It is approximately two fingers wide at its teno-osseous insertion. The tendon feels bony to palpation.

The subscapularis bursa lies deep to the tendon in front of the neck of the scapula and usually communicates with the joint capsule of the shoulder. It is always extremely tender to palpation.

Technique

- *Patient sits supported with arm by side and held in 45° lateral rotation.*
- *Identify coracoid process anteriorly. Move laterally, and feel small protuberance of lesser tuberosity by passively rotating arm.*
- *Insert needle at mid point of tuberosity angling slightly laterally. Touch bone close to insertion.*
- *Pepper solution into teno-osseous junction of tendon or deposit bolus deep to tendon into bursa.*

Aftercare

Relative rest for one week then progressive stretching and strengthening programme when pain free.

Comments

Subscapularis bursitis and tendonitis are often difficult to differentiate. The bursa is implicated if there is more pain on the scarf test than on resisted medial rotation, and if there is even more than usual tenderness to palpation. They are often inflamed together and then both can be infiltrated at the same time by peppering the tendon first and then going through it to inflate the bursa.

30

SUBSCAPULARIS TENDON AND BURSA

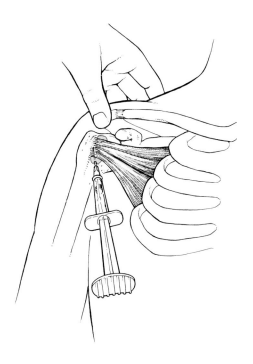

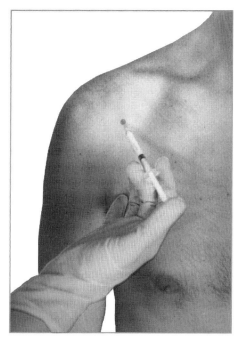

Chronic bursitis

Cause

Overuse.

Findings

Pain in deltoid area.
Painful: passive elevation and medial rotation;
    resisted abduction and lateral rotation, often on release of resistance;
    arc on active abduction.

Equipment

SYRINGE	NEEDLE	KENALOG 40	LOCAL ANAESTHETIC
5 ml	21G 1.5" (0.8 × 40 mm)	20 mg	4.5 ml 1%

Anatomy

The bursa lies mainly under the acromion, but it is very variable in size and there may be more than one. Occasionally a tender area can be palpated around the edge of the acromion.

Technique

- *Patient sits with arm hanging by side to distract humerus from acromion.*
- *Identify lateral edge of acromion.*
- *Insert needle at mid point of acromion and angle slightly upwards under acromion to full length.*
- *Slowly withdraw needle while simultaneously injecting fluid in a bolus wherever there is no resistance. Sometimes a swelling caused by the fluid is visible around the edge of the acromion.*

Aftercare

Relief of pain after one injection is usual but the patient must be advised to maintain correct posture with retraction and depression of the shoulders and to avoid elevation of the arm above the shoulder for one week. After this the patient commences resisted lateral rotation and retraction exercises and retraining of overarm activities in order to avoid recurrence.

Comments

This is the most common injectable lesion found in musculoskeletal medicine (See Appendix). Results are usually excellent but the exercise programme must be maintained to prevent recurrence. In long-standing bursitis there is often loculation of the bursa. In this case resistance will be felt while injecting the solution, so the needle must be fanned around under the acromion in order to inject separate pockets of the bursa. The sensation is that of trying to inject a sponge.

Occasionally calcification occurs within the bursa and hard resistance is felt. Infiltration with a large bore needle and local anaesthetic may be helpful. Failing this, surgical clearance is recommended.

SUBDELTOID BURSA

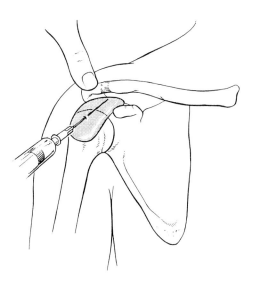

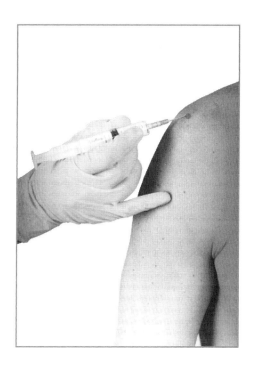

Acute or chronic capsulitis

Cause

Trauma.
Occasionally overuse, e.g. fencing.

Findings

Pain in elbow joint.
Painful passive limitation of: *more* flexion;
                                     less extension.

Equipment

SYRINGE	NEEDLE	KENALOG 40	LOCAL ANAESTHETIC
5 ml	25G 1″ (0.5 × 25 mm)	20 mg	5 ml 1%

Anatomy

The capsule of the elbow joint contains all three joints – the radio-humeral, radio-ulnar and humero-ulnar. The posterior approach above the top of the head of the radius is the safest and easiest.

Technique

■ *Patient sits with elbow supported at 45° of flexion.*

■ *Identify head of radius posteriorly and space between it and humerus.*

■ *Insert needle parallel to the top of the head of radius and penetrate capsule.*

■ *Deposit solution in a bolus.*

Aftercare

After a couple of days the patient should start increasing range of motion within the limits of pain.

Comments

This is not a very common injection. If the cause of the symptoms is one or more loose bodies within the joint, the treatment is mobilization under strong traction. If the range is improved by this but the pain persists, an injection may be considered.

34

ELBOW JOINT

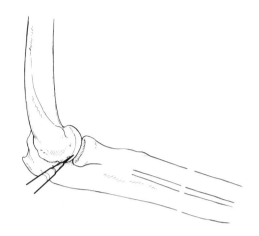

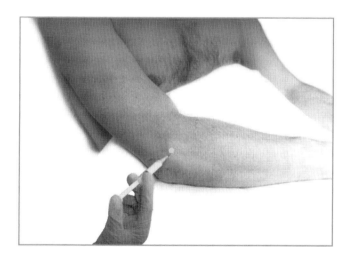

COMMON EXTENSOR TENDON

Chronic tendonitis — 'Tennis Elbow'

Cause

Overuse.

Findings

Pain at lateral aspect of elbow.
Painful resisted extension of the wrist with elbow extended.

Equipment

SYRINGE	NEEDLE	KENALOG 40	LOCAL ANAESTHETIC
1 ml	25G 0.5″ (0.33 × 13 mm)	10 mg	0.75 ml 2%

Anatomy

Tennis elbow occurs most commonly at the teno-osseous origin of the common extensor tendon at the elbow. The tendon arises from the anterior facet of the lateral epicondyle which is approximately the size of the little finger nail. The facet faces anterio-laterally.

Technique

- *Patient sits with supported elbow bent at right angle and forearm supinated to relax the tendon.*
- *Identify facet lying anteriorly on lateral epicondyle.*
- *Insert needle in line with cubital crease perpendicular to the facet until it touches bone.*
- *Pepper solution into tendon.*

Aftercare

It is essential that the patient rests for at least 10 days. Any lifting or carrying must be done only with the palm facing upward so that the flexors rather than the extensors are used. After about a week, stretching of the extensors is begun and a strengthening programme started when resisted extension is pain free. If the case was a racket sport, the weight, handle size and stringing of the racket should be checked as well as the stroke technique.

Comments

Although the teno-osseous junction is the most common site, the lesion can occur in the body of the tendon, in the muscle belly and at the origin of the extensor carpi radialis longus. It is important to ignore tender trigger points in the body of the tendon, which are present in everyone, and to place the needle exactly at the very small site of the lesion.

One injection in the correct place usually suffices, but if the symptoms recur, a second injection is given followed by strong deep friction and Mill's manipulation a few days later. Alternatively, sclerosant injection can be used. Failing all these approaches, tenotomy may be performed although this is rarely necessary. Depigmentation and subcutaneous atrophy may occur on thin females.

36

COMMON EXTENSOR TENDON

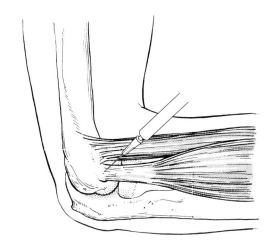

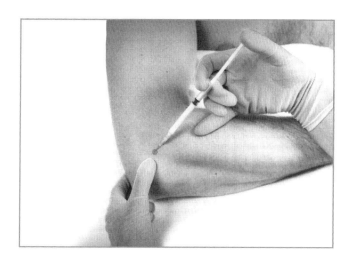

Chronic tendonitis — 'Golfer's Elbow'

Cause

Overuse.

Findings

Pain at medial aspect of elbow.
Painful: resisted flexion of wrist;
        occasional resisted pronation.

Equipment

SYRINGE	NEEDLE	KENALOG 40	LOCAL ANAESTHETIC
1 ml	25G 0.5" (0.33 × 13 mm)	10 mg	0.75 ml 2%

Anatomy

The common flexor tendon at the elbow arises from the anterior facet on the medial epicondyle. It is approximately the size of the little finger nail at its teno-osseous origin.

Technique

- *Patient sits with supported arm extended.*

- *Identify anterior facet on medial epicondyle.*

- *Insert needle perpendicular to facet and touch bone.*

- *Pepper solution into tendon.*

Aftercare

Relative rest for one week then stretching and strengthening exercises.

Comments

Occasionally the lesion occurs at the musculo-tendinous junction. Infiltration at this point may not be as effective but electrotherapy and deep friction can be successful.

COMMON FLEXOR TENDON

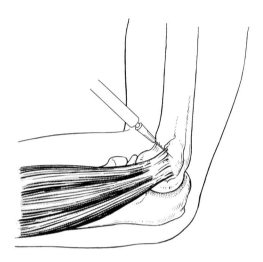

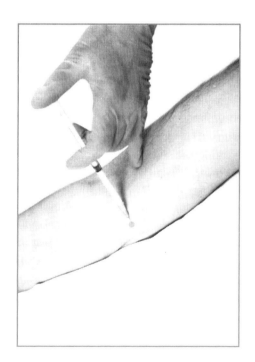

BICEPS TENDON INSERTION

Chronic tendonitis or bursitis

Cause

Overuse.

Findings

Pain at front of elbow.
Painful: resisted flexion and supination;
          passive extension and pronation if bursa affected.

Equipment

SYRINGE	NEEDLE	KENALOG 40	LOCAL ANAESTHETIC
TENDON 1 ml BURSA 2 ml	23G 1.25" (0.6 × 30 mm)	TENDON 10 mg BURSA 20 mg	TENDON 0.75 ml 2% BURSA 2 ml 1%

Anatomy

Although the biceps can be affected at any point along its length, the most commonly affected site is as it inserts into the radial tuberosity on the antero-medial aspect of the shaft of the radius. A small bursa lies at this point and can also be inflamed together with the tendon or on its own.

The insertion of the biceps can be identified by following the path of the tendon distal to the cubital crease while the patient resists elbow flexion. The patient then relaxes the muscle and the tuberosity can be palpated on the ulnar side of the radius while passively pronating and supinating the forearm. The site is always very tender to palpation.

Technique

- *Patient lies face down with arm extended and palm flat down on table. Passively pronate forearm fully while keeping humerus still.*

- *Identify radial tuberosity two fingers distal to radial head.*

- *Insert needle perpendicular to touch bone.*

- *Pepper solution into tendon or bolus into bursa, or both as necessary.*

Aftercare

Rest for one week before beginning graded strengthening and stretching routine.

Comments

Differentiation between bursitis and tendonitis is often difficult. If there is more pain on passive flexion and pronation than on resisted flexion, and extreme sensitivity to palpation, the bursa is more suspect. If in doubt, infiltrate the bursa first and assess a week later.

BICEPS TENDON INSERTION

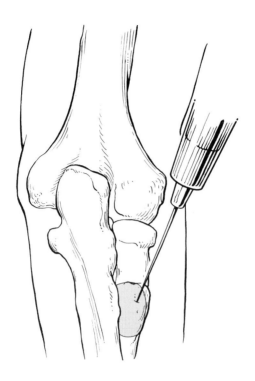

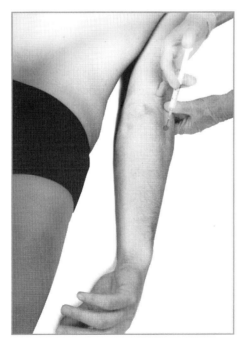

OLECRANON BURSA

Acute or chronic bursitis

Cause

Sustained compression or fall/direct blow onto elbow.

Findings

Pain at posterior aspect of elbow joint.
Painful: passive flextion and sometimes extension;
      resisted extension.
Tender area over bursa and occasionally obvious swelling.

Equipment

SYRINGE	NEEDLE	KENALOG 40	LOCAL ANAESTHETIC
2 ml	23G 1.25" (0.6 × 30 mm)	20 mg	2 ml 1%

Anatomy

The bursa lies at the posterior aspect of the elbow and is approximately the size of a golf ball.

Technique

- Patient sits with supported elbow at right angle.

- Identify centre of tender area of bursa.

- Insert needle into central area.

- Deposit solution into bursa in a bolus.

Aftercare

Relative rest for a week then resumption of normal activities avoiding leaning on elbow.

Comments

Occasionally a direct blow or fall may cause haemorrhagic bursitis when the treatment should be immediate aspiration of all blood prior to the infiltration. Aspiration is always done first and if blood or suspicious fluid is withdrawn, infiltration should not be given at the same time.

OLECRANON BURSA

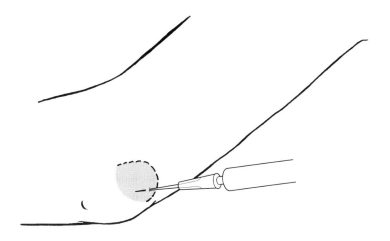

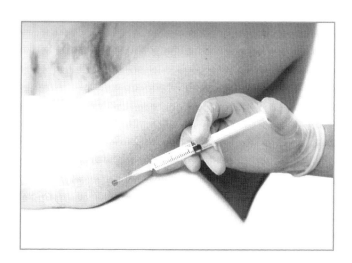

Acute capsulitis

Cause

Rheumatoid arthritis.

Findings

Pain in wrist joint.
Equal painful limitation of passive extension and flexion.

Equipment

SYRINGE	NEEDLE	KENALOG 40	LOCAL ANAESTHETIC
2 ml	23G 1.25" (0.6 × 30 mm)	20 mg	1.5 ml 1%

Anatomy

The wrist joint capsule is not continuous and has septa dividing it into separate compartments. For this reason it cannot be injected at one spot.

Technique

- *Patient places hand palm down.*

- *Identify mid carpus proximal to hollow dip of capitate.*

- *Insert needle at mid point of carpus.*

- *Deposit solution at different points across the dorsum of the wrist both into the ligaments and also intracapsular where possible.*

Aftercare

The patient rests in a splint until the pain subsides and then begins gentle mobilizing exercises within the pain free range.

Comments

This is not a common area for injection except in the patient with rheumatoid arthritis. Patients with other causes such as trauma, overuse or osteoarthritis usually respond well to a short period of electrotherapy and rest followed by passive and active mobilization techniques.

WRIST JOINT

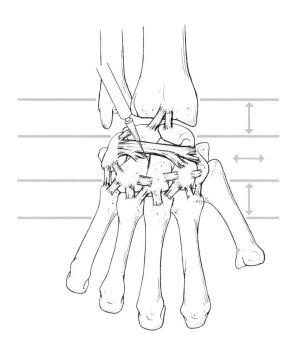

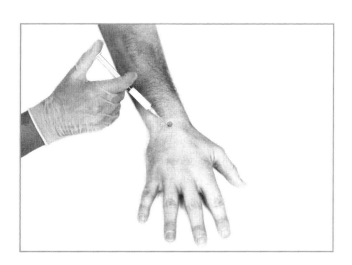

Chronic capsulitis

Cause

Osteoarthritis or rheumatoid arthritis.
Trauma.

Findings

Pain at end of forearm.
Painful: passive pronation and supination at end range.

Equipment

SYRINGE	NEEDLE	KENALOG 40	LOCAL ANAESTHETIC
2 ml	25G 5/8″ (0.33 × 20 mm)	10 mg	1.5 ml 1%

Anatomy

The inferior radio-ulnar joint is about a finger's width in length and includes the triangular cartilage which separates the ulnar from the carpus. With the palm facing downwards, the joint lies one third across the wrist just medial to the bump of the end of the ulnar. The joint line is identified by gliding the ends of the radius and ulnar against each other.

Technique

- *Patient places hand palm down.*

- *Identify joint line.*

- *Insert needle perpendicular and penetrate capsule.*

- *Deposit solution in bolus.*

Aftercare

Rest for one week.

Comments

Tears of the cartilage are quite common, especially after trauma or fracture. In this case pain is found on full passive supination and flexion, and on resisted flexion in ulnar deviation. The most pain provoking test is the grind test – compressing the wrist into ulnar deviation and scooping it in a semi-circular movement towards flexion. The patient often complains of painful clicking and occasionally the wrist locks. Mobilization helps relieve the pain but an injection can be given in the acute phase.

INFERIOR RADIO-ULNAR JOINT

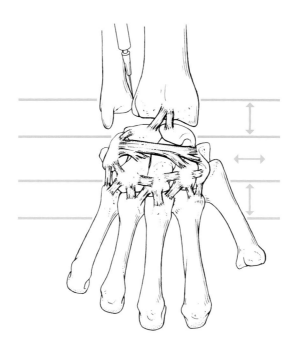

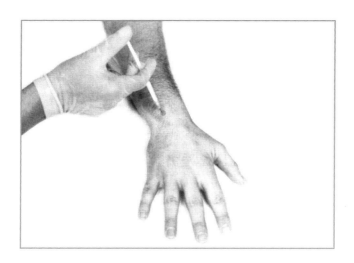

Acute or chronic capsulitis

Cause

Overuse or trauma.

Findings

Thumb: painful passive adduction of thumb backwards behind hand;
painful loss of passive extension.
Fingers: painful loss of passive flexion at interphalangeal joints;
painful loss of passive extension at distal phalangeal joints.

Equipment

SYRINGE	NEEDLE	KENALOG 40	LOCAL ANAESTHETIC
1 ml	25G 0.5" (0.33 × 13 mm)	THUMB 10 mg FINGERS 5 mg	THUMB 0.75 ml 2% FINGERS 0.5 ml 2%

Anatomy

The first metacarpal articulates with the trapezium. The easiest entry site is at the apex of the snuff box on the dorsum of the wrist. The joint line is found by passively flexing and extending the thumb while palpating for the joint space between the two bones.

The distal thumb and finger joints can best be infiltrated from the medial or lateral aspect at the joint line.

Technique

- *Patient rests hand in mid position with thumb up.*

- *Identify gap of joint space between metacarpal to trapezium.*

- *Insert needle into gap.*

- *Deposit solution in a bolus.*

Aftercare

Patient begins gentle active and passive mobilizing exercise within the pain free range and is advised against overuse of the thumb or fingers. Dipping the fingers into warm wax baths and using the wax ball as an exercise tool is beneficial.

Comments

Trapezio-metacarpal joint capsulitis is a common lesion of older females and the results of infiltration are uniformly excellent. Often it is several years before a repeat injection is required provided the patient does not grossly overuse the joint.

Infiltrating the finger joints can be difficult and sometimes it is necessary to anaesthetize the capsule with some of the solution while trying to enter the joint.

THUMB JOINT

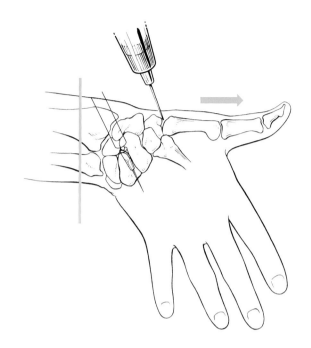

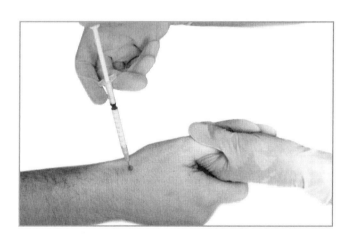

De Quervain's tendonitis of abductor pollicis longus and extensor pollicis brevis

Cause

Overuse.

Findings

Pain over base of thumb and over styloid process of radius.
Painful: resisted abduction and extension of thumb;
              passive flexion of thumb across palm.

Equipment

SYRINGE	NEEDLE	KENALOG 40	LOCAL ANAESTHETIC
1 ml	25G 0.5" (0.33 × 13 mm)	5–10 mg	0.75 ml 2%

Anatomy

The abductor pollicis longus and extensor pollicis brevis usually run together in a single sheath on the radial side of the wrist. The styloid process is always tender so comparison should be made with the pain free side. The two tendons can often be seen when the thumb is held in extension, or can be palpated at the base of the metacarpal.

The aim is to slide the needle between the two tendons and deposit the solution within the sheath.

Technique

- *Patient places hand vertical with thumb held in slight flexion.*
- *Identify gap betwen the two tendons.*
- *Insert needle into gap then slide proximally between the tendons.*
- *Deposit solution as bolus within tendon sheath.*

Aftercare

Rest for a week followed by avoidance of the provoking activity and strengthening regime.

Comments

Provided the wrist is not too swollen, a small sausage shape can be seen where the solution distends the tendon sheath.

This is an area where depigmentation or subcutaneous atrophy can occur, especially on thin females. Although recovery can take place, the results may be permanent. The patient should be warned of this possibility.

THUMB TENDONS

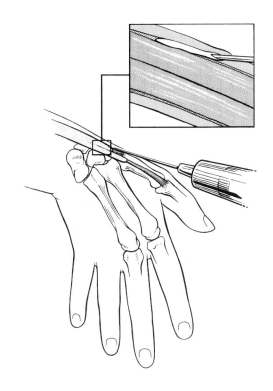

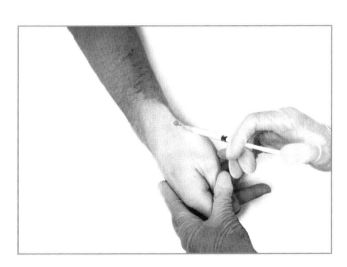

Trigger finger

Cause

Spontaneous onset.

Findings

Painful clicking and sometimes locking of a finger with inability to extend. A tender nodule can be palpated, usually at the base of the finger.

Equipment

SYRINGE	NEEDLE	KENALOG 40	LOCAL ANAESTHETIC
1 ml	25G 0.5″ (0.33 × 13 mm)	10 mg	1 ml 2%

Anatomy

Trigger finger is caused by enlargement of a nodule within the flexor tendon sheath.

Technique

- *Patient places hand palm up.*
- *Identify nodule.*
- *Insert needle into nodule.*
- *Deposit solution in a bolus.*

Aftercare

No particular restriction is placed on the patient's activities.

Comments

This injection is universally effective. Although the nodule usually remains, it can continue asymptomatic indefinitely.

52

FLEXOR TENDON NODULE

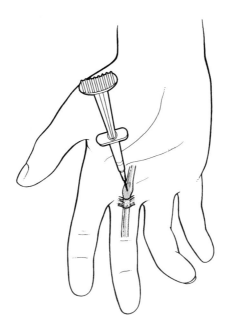

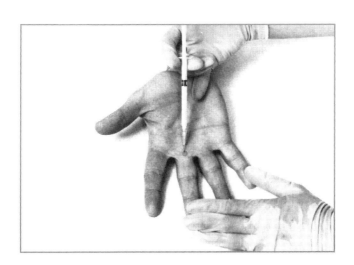

Median nerve compression under flexor retinaculum

Cause

Overuse or trauma.
Pregnancy, hypothyroidism, rheumatoid arthritis.
Idiopathic.

Findings

Pins and needles in the distribution of the median nerve, especially at night.
It is sometimes possible to reproduce the pins and needles by tapping the median
nerve at the wrist (Tinnel's sign) or by holding the wrist in full flexion for 30
seconds and then releasing (Phalen's sign).

Equipment

SYRINGE	NEEDLE	KENALOG 40	LOCAL ANAESTHETIC
1 ml	23G 1.25″ (0.6 × 30 mm)	20 mg	–

Anatomy

The flexor retinaculum of the wrist attaches to four sites: the pisiform and the
scaphoid; the hook of hamate and the trapezium. It is approximately as wide as the
thumb and the proximal edge lies at the distal wrist crease.

The median nerve lies immediately under the palmaris longus tendon at the
mid-point of the wrist, and medial to the flexor carpi radialis tendon. Not every
patient will have a palmaris longus present.

Technique

- *Patient places hand palm up.*
- *Identify flexor carpi radialis tendon lying on radial side of wrist by resisting wrist flexion.*
- *Insert needle at 45° at proximal wrist crease just medial to flexor carpi radialis tendon. Slide distally until the needle point lies under the mid-point of the retinaculum.*
- *Deposit solution in bolus.*

Aftercare

The patient rests for a few days and then resumes normal activities. A night splint
is often helpful in the early stages after the infiltration.

Comments

Care should be taken to avoid inserting the needle too vertically, when it will go
into bone, or too horizontally, when it will enter the retinaculum. If the patient
experiences pins and needles, the needle is repositioned. Although one injection is
often successful, recurrences are common. Further injections can be given if some
relief was obtained, but if the symptoms still recur surgery may be required.

CARPAL TUNNEL

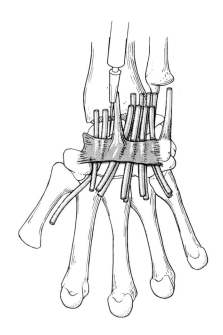

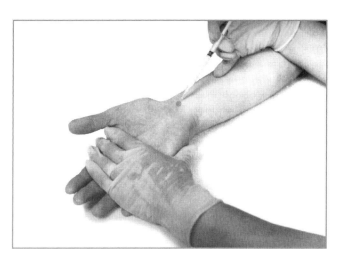

Acute capsulitis

Cause

Osteoarthritis with night pain and radiating pain which is no longer responding to physiotherapy.

Findings

Buttock, groin or anterior thigh pain.
Painful limitation *mostly* of passive medial rotation, then flexion, abduction and extension.
Hard endfeel on passive testing.

Equipment

SYRINGE	NEEDLE	KENALOG 40	LOCAL ANAESTHETIC
10 ml	21G 3" (0.8 × 75 mm)	30 TO 40 mg	8–10 ml 0.5%

Anatomy

The hip joint capsule attaches to the base of the surgical neck of the femur. Therefore, if the needle is inserted to the neck, the solution will be deposited within the capsule. The safest and easiest approach is from the lateral aspect.

The greater trochanter is triangular in shape with a sharp angulation of the apex overhanging the neck. This part is difficult to palpate, especially on patients with excessive adipose tissue, so allow a little extra above the most prominent part of the trochanter. Deep pressure is necessary to feel the upper edge.

Technique

- *Patient lies on pain free side with lower leg flexed and upper leg straight and resting on pillow so that it lies horizontal.*
- *Identify greater trochanter with finger while passively abducting patient's upper leg.*
- *Insert needle perpendicular to skin about a finger's width proximal to trochanter until it touches the neck of femur. There is usually no sensation of penetrating the capsule.*
- *Deposit solution in a bolus.*

Aftercare

Patient gradually increases pain free activity but limits weight-bearing exercise.

Comments

The lateral approach to the hip joint is both simple and safe. It is not necessary to do the technique under fluoroscopy and the procedure is not particularly painful. This injection is usually given to patients who are on a waiting list for surgery. It is successful in giving temporary pain relief and can, if necessary, be repeated at intervals of no less than three months. An annual X-ray monitors degenerative change.

HIP JOINT

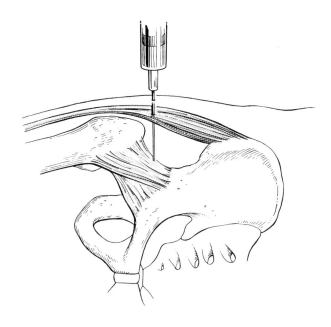

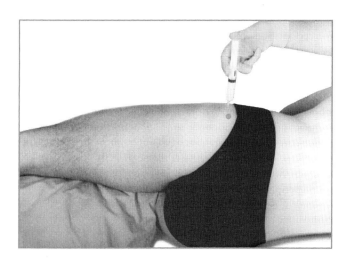

ADDUCTOR TENDONS

Chronic tendonitis

Cause

Overuse or trauma.

Findings

Pain in groin.
Painful: resisted adduction;
passive abduction.

Equipment

SYRINGE	NEEDLE	KENALOG 40	LOCAL ANAESTHETIC
2 ml	23G 1.25" (0.6 × 30 mm)	20 mg	1.5 ml 1%

Anatomy

The adductor tendons arise from the pubis and are approximately two fingers wide at their origin. The lesion can lie at the teno-osseous junction or in the body of the tendon. The technique described is for the more common site at the teno-osseous junction.

Technique

- *The patient lies supine with leg slightly abducted and laterally rotated.*
- *Identify the origin of the tendon.*
- *Insert needle into tendon angled towards bone of pubis and touch bone.*
- *Pepper solution into teno-osseous junction.*

Aftercare

Rest for one week then graduated stretching and strengthening programme.

Comments

For the less common site at the body of the tendon, the solution is peppered into the tender area in the body, but deep friction and stretching is often more effective here.

ADDUCTOR TENDONS

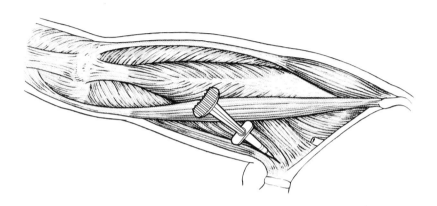

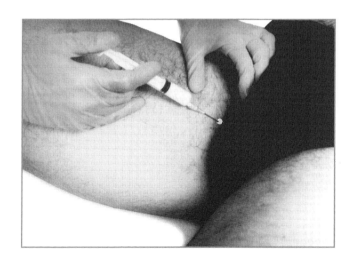

Chronic tendonitis or acute or chronic ischial bursitis

Cause

Overuse, such as prolonged riding on horse or bicycle, or running.
Trauma: fall onto buttock.

Findings

Pain in buttock.
Painful: resisted extension;
        passive straight leg raise.
Very tender over ischial tuberosity.

Equipment

SYRINGE	NEEDLE	KENALOG 40	LOCAL ANAESTHETIC
TENDON 2 ml BURSA 5 ml	21G 2″ (0.8 × 50 mm)	TENDON 20 mg BURSA 20 mg	TENDON 1.5 ml 1% BURSA 4 ml 1%

Anatomy

The hamstrings have a common origin arising from the ischial tuberosity. The tendon is approximately three fingers wide here. The ischial bursa lies between the gluteus maximus and the bone of the ischial tuberosity. It is approximately the size of a small orange.

Technique

- *Patient lies on good side with lower leg straight and upper leg flexed.*
- *Identify ischial tuberosity and tendon lying immediately distal.*
- *Insert needle into mid point of tendon and angle up toward tuberosity to touch bone.*
- *Pepper solution into teno-osseous junction or deposit in bolus into bursa.*

Aftercare

Avoidance of precipitating activities such as sitting on hard surfaces or prolonged running is maintained for about a week and then graduated stretching and strengthening programme is started.

Comments

Tendonitis and bursitis may occur together at this site, in which case a larger volume is drawn up and both lesions infiltrated. As usual, it is difficult to differentiate between the two lesions, but if there is a history of a fall or friction overuse, and there is extreme tenderness at the tuberosity, bursitis is suspected.

Occasionally haemorrhagic bursitis can occur as a result of a hard fall or blow. Aspiration of the blood is then performed.

60

HAMSTRING TENDON ORIGIN

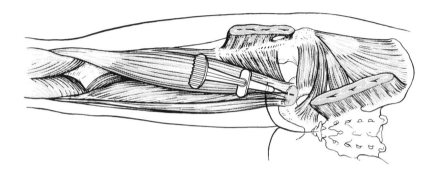

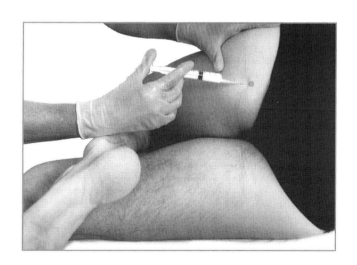

Chronic bursitis

Cause

Overuse.

Findings

Pain and tenderness over the upper lateral quadrant of the buttock.
Painful: passive flexion, abduction and adduction;
        resisted abduction and extension.

Equipment

SYRINGE	NEEDLE	KENALOG 40	LOCAL ANAESTHETIC
10–20 ml	21G 3″ (0.8 × 75 mm)	20 mg	10–20 ml 0.5%

Anatomy

The gluteal bursae are variable in number, size and shape. They can be found deep to the gluteal muscles on the blade of the ilium and also between the layers of the three gluteal muscles. The painful area guides the placement of the needle but comparison between the two sides is essential as this area is always tender.

Technique

- *Patient lies on unaffected side with lower leg extended and upper leg flexed.*

- *Identify centre of tender area in upper outer quadrant of buttock.*

- *Insert needle perpendicular to skin until it touches blade of ilium.*

- *Deposit fluid in areas of no resistance while moving needle in a circular manner out towards surface – imagine the needle walking up a spiral staircase.*

Aftercare

The patient must avoid overusing the leg for a week and can then gradually resume normal activities.

Comments

There are no major blood vessels or nerves in the area of the bursae so the injection is safe. Feeling for a loss of resistance within the gluteus minor and maximus guides the clinician in depositing the fluid.

62

GLUTEAL BURSA

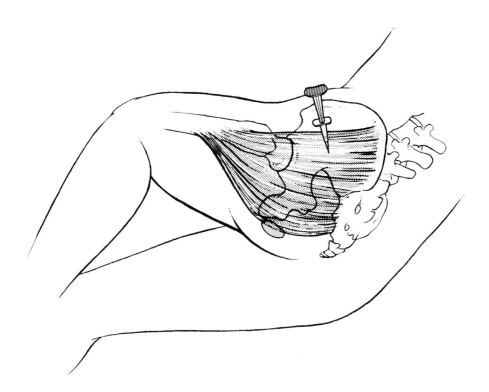

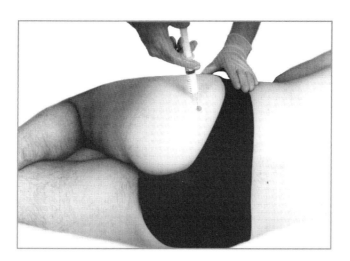

PSOAS BURSA

Chronic bursitis

Cause

Overuse, especially sports or activities involving repeated hip flexion movements, e.g. hurdling, ballet, javelin throwing, football.

Findings

Pain in groin.
Painful: passive flexion, adduction, abduction and possibly extension;
resisted flexion and adduction;
psoas compression test — semicircular compression of femur from full flexion to adduction.

Equipment

SYRINGE	NEEDLE	KENALOG 40	LOCAL ANAESTHETIC
10 ml	21G 3″ (0.8 × 75 mm)	20 mg	8–10 ml 0.5%

Anatomy

The psoas bursa lies between the psoas tendon and the anterior aspect of the neck of the femur. It also lies deep to the three major vessels in the groin — the femoral vein, artery and nerve. For this reason, correct placement of the needle is essential. It is approximately the size of a small orange.

Technique

- *Patient lies supine.*
- *Identify femoral pulse at mid-point of inguinal ligament. Move three fingers distally and three fingers laterally. The entry point lies in direct line with the anterior superior iliac spine and is on the edge of the sartorius muscle.*
- *Insert needle at this point and angle 45° cephalad and 45° medially. Visualize the needle sliding under the three major vessels towards the anterior aspect of the neck of femur.*
- *When the needle touches bone, withdraw slightly and deposit solution in bolus deep to tendon.*

Aftercare

Absolute avoidance of the activities which irritated the bursa must be maintained for at least a week, then a stretching of hip extension and muscle balancing programme is initiated.

Comments

Although this injection may appear intimidiating to the clinician at the first attempt, the approach outlined above is safe and effective. Very rarely it is possible to catch a lateral branch of the fermoral nerve and temporarily anaesthetize the quadriceps. It is best to keep well lateral at the insertion point and if the patient complains of a tingling pain to reposition the needle before depositing solution.

PSOAS BURSA

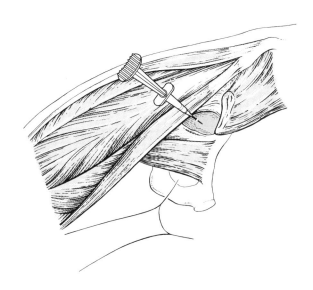

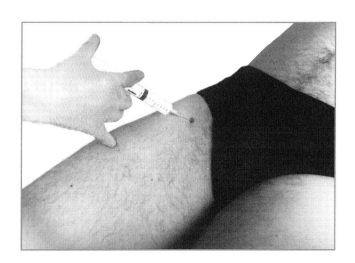

TROCHANTERIC BURSA

Acute or chronic bursitis

Cause

Usually a direct blow or fall onto hip.
Occasionally overuse.

Findings

Pain and tenderness over greater trochanter.
Painful: passive abduction, adduction and possibly flexion and extension;
        resisted abduction.

Equipment

SYRINGE	NEEDLE	KENALOG 40	LOCAL ANAESTHETIC
2 ml	23G 1.25" (0.6 × 30 mm)	20 mg	1.5 ml 1%

Anatomy

The trochanteric bursa lies over the greater trochanter of the femur. It is approximately the size of a golf ball.

Technique

- *Patient lies on unaffected side with lower leg flexed and upper leg extended.*

- *Identify tender area over greater trochanter.*

- *Insert needle at centre of tender area and touch bone of greater trochanter.*

- *Deposit solution by feeling for area of lack of resistance and introduce fluid there.*

Aftercare

Avoidance of overuse for a week and then gradual return to normal activity.

Comments

A fall or direct blow onto the trochanter can cause a haemorrhagic bursitis. This calls for immediate aspiration of the blood.

66

TROCHANTERIC BURSA

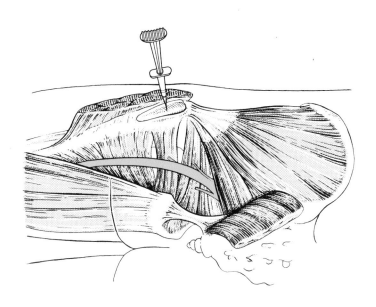

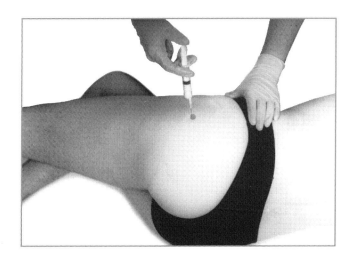

KNEE JOINT

Acute or chronic capsulitis

Cause

Osteoarthritis or rheumatoid arthritis.
Trauma.

Findings

Pain in knee joint.
Painful and limited: passive flexion *more* than extension with hard end feel.
Possible effusion.

Equipment

SYRINGE	NEEDLE	KENALOG 40	LOCAL ANAESTHETIC
10 ml	23G 1.25″ (0.6 × 30 mm)	20–30 mg	8–9 ml 0.5%

Anatomy

There are several ways to infiltrate the knee joint. The easiest and safest is the medial approach under the patella. Once the needle point is behind the patella it must be intra-articular and fat pads and the menisci are avoided. There is more space medial to patella as the femoral condyle is smaller.

Technique

- *Patient sits with knee supported.*

- *Place thumb on lateral side of relaxed patella and push medially.*

- *Identify medial edge of patella while maintaining position with thumb.*

- *Insert needle horizontally at mid point of medial edge of patella between it and the femoral condyle and slide under patella.*

- *Deposit solution as bolus.*

Aftercare

The patient avoids undue weight-bearing activity for about a week and then is given strengthening and mobilizing exercises to continue at home.

Comments

The same approach can be used whether infiltrating or aspirating fluid or blood.

The injection will give temporary relief from pain and provided the knee is not overused this can last for some time. Repeat injections can be given at intervals of not less than three months with an annual X-ray to monitor joint degeneration.

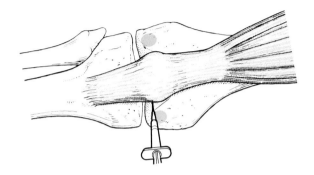

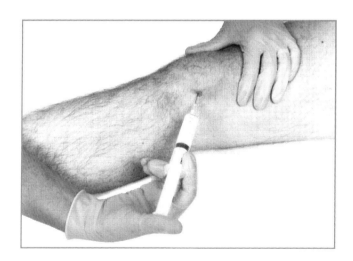

SUPERIOR TIBIO-FIBULAR JOINT

Acute or chronic capsulitis

Cause

Usually trauma such as a fall with forced medial rotation of the foot with a flexed knee.

Findings

Pain over joint.
Painful: resisted flexion of knee;
          full passive medial rotation of knee.

Equipment

SYRINGE	NEEDLE	KENALOG 40	LOCAL ANAESTHETIC
2 ml	23G 1.25" (0.6 × 30 mm)	20 mg	1.5 ml 1%

Anatomy

The superior tibio-fibular joint lies on the lateral aspect of the knee. The joint line runs medially from superior to inferior. The anterior approach to the joint is safer as the peroneal nerve lies posterior.

Technique

■ *Identify the head of the fibula and the joint line medial to it.*

■ *Insert needle at midpoint of joint line and aim obliquely laterally to penetrate capsule.*

■ *Deposit solution in bolus.*

Aftercare

Relative rest for about a week and then resumption of normal activities.
   Strengthening of the biceps femoris may be necessary.

Comments

Occasionally the joint is subluxed and has to be manipulated before infiltration.
   The unstable joint can be treated with sclerotherapy.

SUPERIOR TIBIO-FIBULAR JOINT

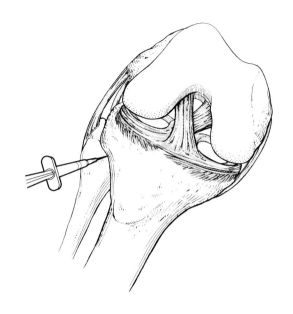

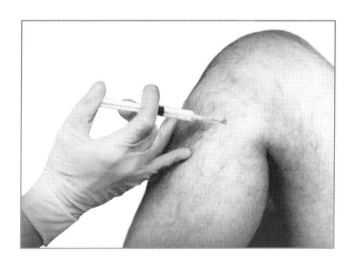

CORONARY LIGAMENT

Ligamentous sprain with or without meniscal tear

Cause

Trauma: a strong forced rotation of the knee.

Findings

Pain, usually at medial joint line.
Painful passive lateral rotation (for medical coronary ligament).
Possible painful meniscal tests.

Equipment

SYRINGE	NEEDLE	KENALOG 40	LOCAL ANAESTHETIC
1 ml	25G 1″ (0.5 × 25 mm)	10 mg	0.75 ml 2%

Anatomy

The coronary ligaments are small thin fibrous bands attaching the menisci to the tibial plateaux. The medial ligament is more usually affected. It can be found by placing the foot on the table with the knee at right angles and turning the foot into lateral rotation. This brings the tibial plateau into prominence and the tender area is sought by pressing in and down onto the plateau.

Technique

- *Patient half lies with knee at right angle and planted foot laterally rotated.*
- *Identify tender area on tibial plateau.*
- *Insert needle vertically down onto plateau.*
- *Pepper all along the tender area.*

Aftercare

Early mobilizing exercise to full range of motion without pain is started.

Comments

These ligaments usually respond extremely well to deep friction – it is not uncommon to cure the symptoms in one session. The injection should be kept for where the friction treatment is not available or where the pain is too intense to allow the pressure of the finger.

Tear or subluxation of the meniscus should be treated first by manipulation.

CORONARY LIGAMENT

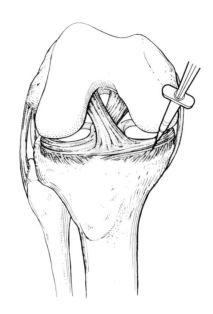

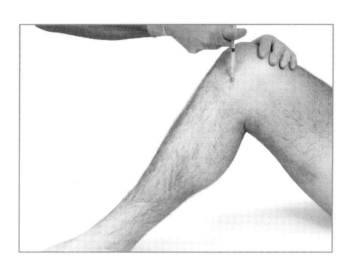

MEDIAL COLLATERAL LIGAMENT

Acute sprain

Cause

Trauma – typically flexion, valgus and lateral rotation of the knee as in a fall while skiing.

Findings

Pain at medial joint line of knee.
Painful: passive valgus;
            passive lateral rotation of the knee.

Equipment

SYRINGE	NEEDLE	KENALOG 40	LOCAL ANAESTHETIC
2 ml	25G 1" (0.5 × 25 mm)	15–20 mg	1.5–2 ml 1%

Anatomy

The medial collateral ligament of the knee runs from the medial condyle of the femur to the medial aspect of the shaft of the tibia and is approximately a hand's width long and a good two fingers wide. It is difficult to palpate the ligament as it is so thin and part of the joint capsule. It is usually sprained at the joint line.

Technique

- *Patient lies with knee supported and slightly flexed.*
- *Identify the medial joint line and tender area of ligament.*
- *Insert needle at mid point of tender area. Do not penetrate right through joint capsule.*
- *Pepper solution along width of ligament in two rows.*

Aftercare

Gentle passive and active movement within the pain free range is started immediately.

Comments

Sprain of this ligament rarely needs to be injected as early physiotherapeutic treatment with ice, massage and mobilization is very effective. The injection approach can be used when this treatment is not available or the patient is in a great deal of pain.

MEDIAL COLLATERAL LIGAMENT

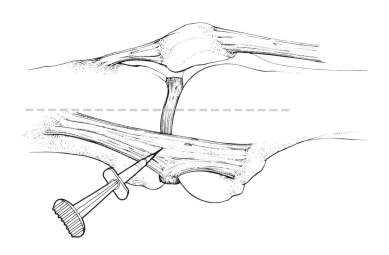

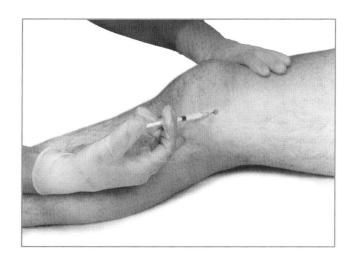

Muscle sprain

Cause

Overuse.

Findings

Pain on superior medial side of patella.
Pain on going down hill or down stairs.
Painful resisted extension of the knee.

Equipment

SYRINGE	NEEDLE	KENALOG 40	LOCAL ANAESTHETIC
2 ml	25G 1" (0.5 × 25 mm)	10 mg	1.5 ml 2%

Anatomy

The quadriceps muscle inserts through an expansion around the borders of the patella. The usual site of the lesion is at the superior medial pole of the patella. This is found by pushing the patella medially with the thumb and palpating up and under the medial edge with a finger to find the tender area.

Technique

- *Patient half lies on table with knee relaxed.*

- *Identify medial edge of superior pole of patella for tender area.*

- *Insert needle horizontally to touch bone of patella.*

- *Pepper solution along line of insertion.*

Aftercare

Patient avoids overusing the knee for at least a week and when pain free begins progressive strengthening and stretching programme.

Comments

This lesion, like the coronary ligament, responds very well to two or three sessions of strong deep friction. The injection is used therefore when the friction is not available, the area is too tender, or to disinflame the expansion prior to friction a week later in a combination approach.

QUADRICEPS EXPANSION

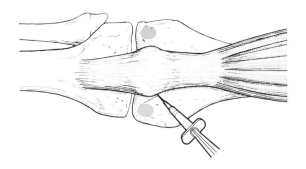

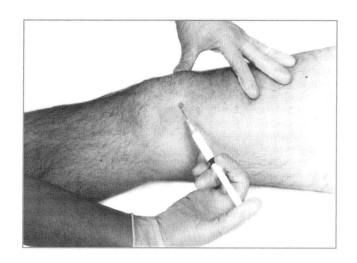

Chronic tendonitis

Cause

Overuse — jumpers and runners.

Findings

Pain at inferior pole of patella.
Painful: resisted extension of knee.

Equipment

SYRINGE	NEEDLE	KENALOG 40	LOCAL ANAESTHETIC
2 ml	23G 1.25″ (0.8 × 30 mm)	20 mg	1.5 ml 1%

Anatomy

The infrapatella tendon arises from the inferior pole of the patella and it is here that it is commonly inflamed. The tendon is at least two fingers wide at its origin.

It is an absolute contraindication to inject corticosteroid *into* the body of the tendon as it is a large, weight-bearing and relatively avascular structure.

Technique

■ *Patient sits with knee supported and extended.*

■ *Place the web of the cephalic index and thumb on superior pole of patella and tilt inferior pole up.*

■ *Identify the tender area at the origin of the tendon on the distal end of the patella.*

■ *Insert needle at mid point of tendon origin at an angle of 45°.*

■ *Pepper solution along tendon in two rows. There should always be some resistance to the needle to ensure that the solution is not being introduced intra-articularly.*

Aftercare

Absolute rest is recommended for at least 10 days before a stretching and strengthening programme is initiated.

Comments

Injecting the origin of the infrapatella tendon at the inferior pole is very safe provided adequate rest is maintained afterwards and that no more than two injections are given in one attack.

In the case of the committed athlete, however, alternative treatment such as deep friction, electrotherapy and taping should be considered.

78

INFRAPATELLA TENDON

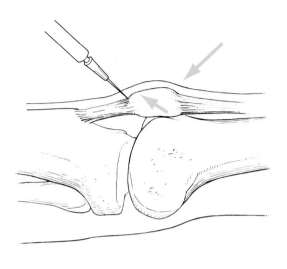

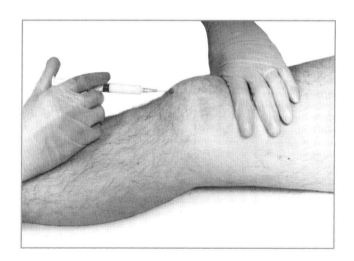

Acute or chronic bursitis

Cause

Overuse – long distance running or prolonged kneeling.
Trauma – direct blow or fall.

Findings

Pain anterior knee below patella.
Painful: resisted extension of knee;
          passive flexion of knee.
Tenderness at mid point of patella tendon.

Equipment

SYRINGE	NEEDLE	KENALOG 40	LOCAL ANAESTHETIC
2 ml	23G 1.25" (0.6 × 30 mm)	20 mg	2 ml 1%

Anatomy

There are two infrapatella bursae – one lies superficial and one deep to the tendon.
The technique described is for the deep bursa which is more commonly affected.

Technique

- *The patient sits with the knee supported in slight flexion.*

- *Identify the tender area at mid point of the tendon.*

- *Insert needle horizontally **behind** tendon from either the medial or lateral side. It is most important that the needle slides in behind the tendon and not into it.*

Aftercare

The patient must avoid all overuse of the knee for at least a week. Where the cause is occupational, such as in carpet layers, a pad with a hole in it to relieve pressure on the bursa should be used.
  Graded stretching and strengthening exercises are then begun.

Comments

It would be tempting to believe that pain found at the mid point of the patella tendon is caused by tendonitis, but in the experience of the authors this is virtually unknown at this site. Infrapatella tendonitis is found consistently at the proximal teno-osseous junction on the patella or rarely at insertion into the tibial tubercle.

INFRAPATELLA BURSA

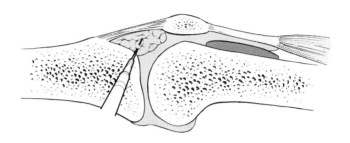

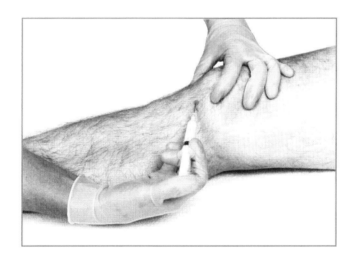

Chronic bursitis

Cause

Overuse – especially dancers or runners.

Findings

Pain at insertion of medial flexors of knee.
Painful: resisted flexion of knee.

Equipment

SYRINGE	NEEDLE	KENALOG 40	LOCAL ANAESTHETIC
2 ml	23G 1.25" (0.6 × 30 mm)	20 mg	2 ml 1%

Anatomy

The pes anseurine is the combined tendon of insertion of the sartorius, gracilis and semi-tendinosus. It attaches on the medial side of the tibia just below the knee joint line. The bursa lies immediately under the tendon and is extremely tender to palpation in the normal knee.

Technique

- *Patient sits with knee supported.*

- *Identify the pes anseurine tendon by making the patient strongly flex the knee against resistance. Follow the combined tendons distally to where they disappear at insertion into tibia. The bursa is found as an area of extreme tenderness deep to the insertion.*

- *Insert needle into centre of area through tendon until it touches bone.*

- *Deposit solution in bolus.*

Aftercare

Avoidance of overuse activities for at least a week when graded stretching and strengthening exercises are started.

Comments

It is important to remember that the bursa is extremely tender to palpation on everybody, so comparison testing must be done on both knees.

PES ANSEURINE BURSA

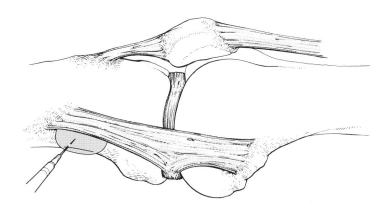

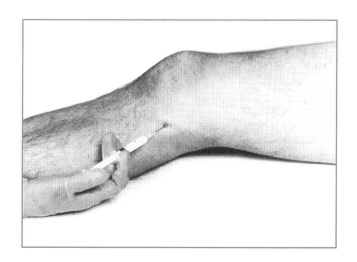

Chronic bursitis

Cause

Overuse – especially long distance runners.

Findings

Pain on the outer side of the knee above the lateral femoral condyle.
Painful: resisted adbuction of leg;
          passive adduction of leg.

Equipment

SYRINGE	NEEDLE	KENALOG 40	LOCAL ANAESTHETIC
2 ml	23G 1.25" (0.6 × 30 mm)	20 mg	1.5 ml 1%

Anatomy

The bursa lies deep to the iliotibial band just above the lateral condyle of the femur.

Technique

■ *Identify the tender area on lateral side of femur.*

■ *Insert needle into bursa passing through tendon to touch bone.*

■ *Deposit solution in bolus.*

Aftercare

Absolute rest must be maintained for about 10 days and then a stretching and strengthening programme initiated.
  Footwear and running technique must be checked and corrected if necessary.

Comments

The lower end of the ilio-tibial tract itself can be irritated but invariably the bursa is also at fault. If both lesions are suspected, both can be infiltrated at the same time.

ILIOTIBIAL BAND BURSA

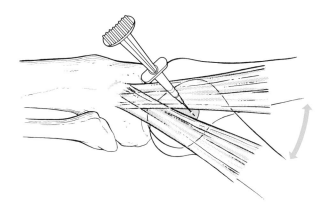

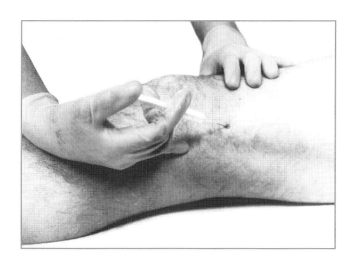

BAKER'S CYST

Cause

Spontaneous insidious onset.

Findings

Obvious swelling in the popliteal fossa – often quite large.

Equipment

SYRINGE	NEEDLE	KENALOG 40	LOCAL ANAESTHETIC
10 OR 20 ml	21G 2" (0.8 × 50 mm)	–	–

Anatomy

Baker's cyst is a sac of synovial fluid caused by seepage through a defect in the posterior wall of the capsule of the knee joint, or by swelling of the semi membranosus bursa.

The popliteal artery and vein, and posterior tibial nerve pass centrally in the popliteal fossa and must be avoided.

Technique

■ *Mark a spot two fingers medial to the midline of the fossa and two fingers below the popliteal crease.*

■ *Insert needle at the marked spot and angle medially at a 45° angle.*

■ *Aspirate at intervals.*

Aftercare

A firm compression bandage can be applied for a day or two.

Comments

If anything other than clear synovial fluid is removed, a specimen should be sent for culture and the appropriate treatment instigated. Invariably the swelling returns within six months to a year.

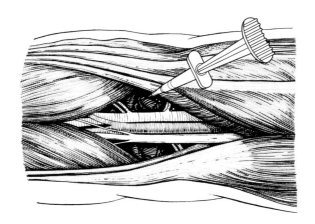

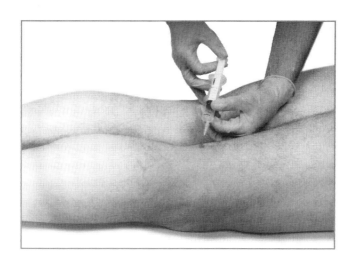

Chronic capsulitis

Cause

Post trauma – previous fracture or severe injury, often many years later.

Findings

Pain at front of ankle.
Painful and limited: *more* passive plantarflexion.
less passive dorsiflexion.

Equipment

SYRINGE	NEEDLE	KENALOG 40	LOCAL ANAESTHETIC
2 ml	23G 1.25" (0.6 × 30 mm)	20 mg	2 ml 1%

Anatomy

The easiest and safest entry point to the ankle joint is at the junction of the tibia and fibula just above the talus. A small triangular space can be palpated there.

Technique

- *Patient lies with foot supported in neutral.*

- *Identify the entry point by passively flexing and extending the ankle while palpating the small triangular space.*

- *Insert needle directly into joint passing through capsule.*

- *Deposit solution as bolus.*

Aftercare

Avoidance of excessive weightbearing activities is maintained for at least a week. The patient should be warned that heavy overuse of the foot will cause a recurrence of symptoms and therefore long distance running should be avoided. Weight control is also advised.

Comments

The ankle joint rarely causes problems except after severe trauma or fracture, and then often many years later. The infiltration is usually very successful in giving long-lasting pain relief and can be repeated if necessary at intervals of at least three months with an annual X-ray to monitor degenerative changes.

ANKLE JOINT

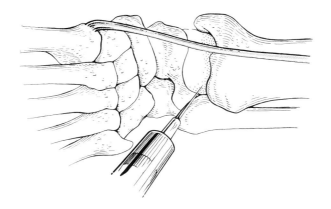

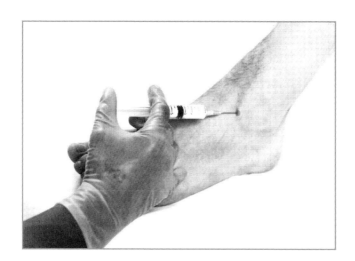

Chronic capsulitis

Cause

Trauma – usually after fracture or severe impaction injury, often many years later. Obesity.

Findings

Pain deep in heel.
Painful and limited: passive adduction of the calcaneus.

Equipment

SYRINGE	NEEDLE	KENALOG 40	LOCAL ANAESTHETIC
2 ml	21G 1.25" (0.6 × 30 mm)	20 mg	1.5 ml 1%

Anatomy

The subtalar joint is divided by an oblique septum into anterior and posterior portions. It is usually slightly easier to enter the joint just above the sustentaculum tali which is a bump of bone lying a thumb's width below the medial malleolus.

Technique

- *Patient lies with foot supported so that medial aspect of heel faces upwards.*

- *Identify sustentaculum tali.*

- *Insert needle immediately above and slightly posterior to sustentaculum tali perpendicular to skin and penetrate capsule.*

- *Deposit half solution here.*

- *Withdraw needle slightly and angle obliquely anteriorly through septum into anterior compartment of joint space and deposit remaining solution here.*

Aftercare

Avoidance of excessive weight-bearing activities for at least a week.
 Orthotics and weight control are helpful in preventing recurrence.

Comments

This is a difficult injection to perform due to the anatomical shape of the joint. It can be repeated at infrequent intervals if necessary.

SUBTALAR JOINT

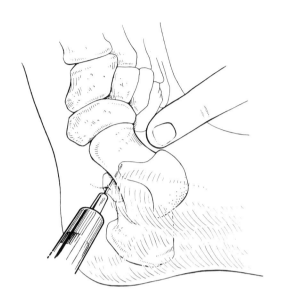

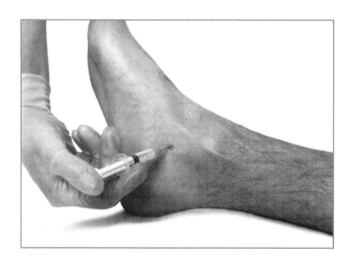

Acute or chronic capsulitis

Cause

Overuse or trauma – female ballet dancers who over point or football players.

Findings

Pain on dorsum of foot – usually at third metatarsal/cuneiform joint line.
Painful limited: adduction and inversion of midtarsal joints.

Equipment

SYRINGE	NEEDLE	KENALOG 40	LOCAL ANAESTHETIC
2 ml	25G 5/8″ (0.5 × 16 mm)	10–15 mg	1–1.5 ml 1%

Anatomy

There are several joints in the mid-tarsus, each with its own capsule. Gross passive testing followed by local joint gliding and palpation should identify the joint involved.

Technique

- *Patient lies with foot supported in neutral.*
- *Identify tender joint line.*
- *Insert needle down into joint space.*
- *Pepper some solution into capsule and remainder as bolus into joint cavity.*

Aftercare

Avoidance of excessive weight-bearing activities for at least a week.

Mobilizing and strengthening exercises and retraining of causal activities follow. Orthotics and weight control if necessary are useful additions.

Comments

This is a universally successful treatment provided sensible attention is paid to aftercare.

MIDTARSAL JOINTS

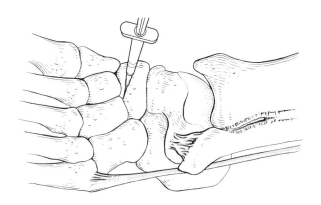

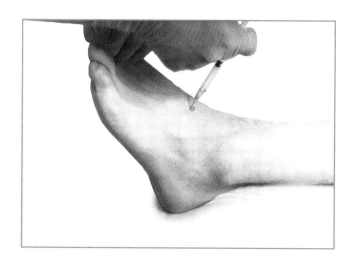

TOE JOINTS

Acute or chronic capsulitis

Cause

Overuse or trauma.
Hallux valgus.

Findings

Pain in toe joint.
Painful limited: flexion of the big toe.

Equipment

SYRINGE	NEEDLE	KENALOG 40	LOCAL ANAESTHETIC
1 ml	25G 5/8" (0.5 × 16 mm)	10 mg	0.75 ml 2%

Anatomy

The first metatarso-phalangeal joint line is most easily found by palpating the space produced at the base of the metacarpal on the dorsal aspect while passively flexing and extending the toe.

Technique

- *Patient lies with foot supported.*

- *Identify and mark joint line and distract big toe with one hand.*

- *Insert needle perpendicular into joint space avoiding the extensor tendon.*

- *Deposit solution as bolus.*

Aftercare

Avoidance of excessive weight-bearing activities for at least a week together with taping of the joint and a toe pad between the toes.

Comments

As with the thumb joint injection, this treatment can be very long-lasting.

The other toe joints are injected from the medial or lateral aspect while under traction.

TOE JOINTS

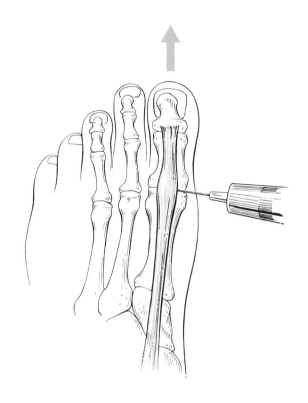

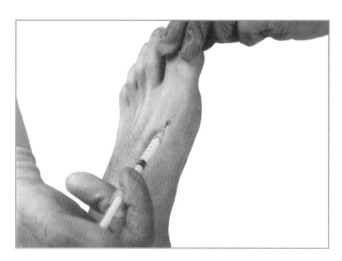

Acute or chronic sprain

Cause

Trauma.
Obesity.
Overpronation of the foot.

Findings

Pain over medial side of foot below medial malleolus.
Painful passive eversion of the ankle in plantarflexion.

Equipment

SYRINGE	NEEDLE	KENALOG 40	LOCAL ANAESTHETIC
1 ml	25G 1" (0.5 × 25 mm)	10 mg	0.5 ml 1%

Anatomy

The deltoid ligament is a strong triangular structure with two layers. It runs from the medial malleolus to the sustentaculum tali on the calcaneum and to the tubercle on the navicular. Sprains here are not as common as at the lateral ligament, but because they do not respond as well to friction and mobilization, injection is worth trying. The inflamed part is usually at the origin on the malleolus.

Technique

■ *Patient sits with medial side of foot accessible.*

■ *Identify lower border of medial malleolus.*

■ *Insert needle upwards to touch bone at midpoint of ligament.*

■ *Pepper solution along attachment to bone.*

Aftercare

To prevent recurrence, the biomechanics of the foot must be carefully checked. Almost always an orthotic is necessary and, in the overweight patient, advice on diet must be given.

Comments

An uncommon but universally successful injection.

DELTOID LIGAMENT

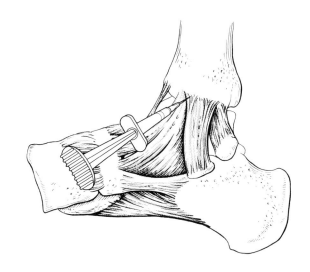

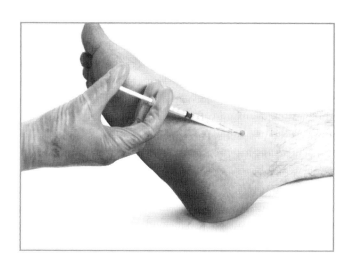

Acute ligamentous sprain

Cause

Inversion injury.

Findings

Pain at lateral side of ankle.
Painful passive inversion of ankle.

Equipment

SYRINGE	NEEDLE	KENALOG 40	LOCAL ANAESTHETIC
1 ml	25G 5/8″ (0.5 × 16 mm)	10 mg	1 ml 2%

Anatomy

The anterior talo-fibular ligament runs medially from the anterior inferior edge of the lateral malleolus to attach to the talus. It is a thin structure and is approximately the width of the little finger.

Technique

- Patient lies supported on table.

- Identify anterior inferior edge of lateral malleolus.

- Insert needle parallel to skin to touch bone.

- Pepper half solution around origin of ligament.

- Turn needle and pepper remainder into insertion on talus.

Aftercare

Patient keeps ankle moving within pain free range. For the first few days ice and taping in eversion may be necessary.

Comments

This lesion responds very well in the acute stage to a regime of ice, elevation, gentle massage, active and passive mobilization and taping. The injection can be used where this treatment is not available or where the pain is acute, but early movement must be encouraged.

LATERAL LIGAMENT

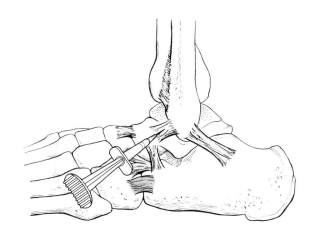

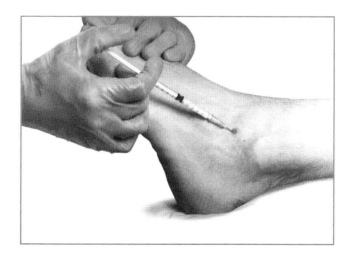

ACHILLES TENDON

Chronic tendonitis

Cause

Overuse.

Findings

Pain at posterior aspect of ankle.
Painful: resisted plantarflexion of the foot.

Equipment

SYRINGE	NEEDLE	KENALOG 40	LOCAL ANAESTHETIC
2 ml	23G 1.25" (0.6 × 30 mm)	20 mg	1.5 ml 1%

Anatomy

The Achilles tendon lies at the end of the gastrocnemius as it inserts into the posterior surface of the calcaneum. *It is absolutely contraindicated* to infiltrate *into* the *body* of the tendon as it is a large, weight-bearing, relatively avascular tendon with a known propensity to rupture.

Technique

- *The patient lies prone with the foot held in dorsiflexion over the end of the bed. This keeps the tendon under tension and facilitates the procedure.*

- *Identify the tender area of the tendon – usually along the sides.*

- *Insert the needle to the medial side and parallel to the tendon.*

- *Slide needle along side of tendon taking care not to enter into the substance of the tendon.*

- *Deposit half the solution while slowly withdrawing needle.*

- *Insert needle to the lateral side of the tendon and repeat procedure with remaining half of the solution.*

Aftercare

Absolute avoidance of any overuse is essential for about 10 days. When pain free, graded stretching and strengthening exercises are begun. Orthotics and retraining in the causal activity are usually necessary.

Comments

Although there are reports of tendon rupture after injection here, this has usually occurred as a result of repeated injections of large dose and volume into the body of the tendon. Depositing the solution along the sides is safe and effective but should not be repeated more than once in one attack. The committed athlete may prefer to receive deep friction at the site instead.

ACHILLES TENDON

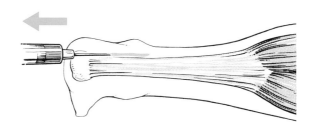

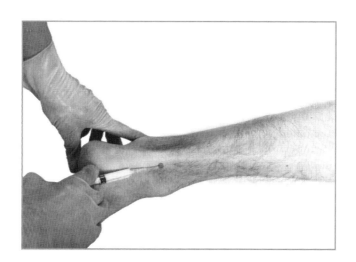

Chronic bursitis

Cause

Overuse – runners and dancers.

Findings

Pain at posterior heel.
Painful: resisted plantarflexion especially at end range;
        full passive plantarflexion.
Tender area anterior to body of achilles tendon.

Equipment

SYRINGE	NEEDLE	KENALOG 40	LOCAL ANAESTHETIC
2 ml	23G 1.25″ (0.6 × 30 mm)	20 mg	1.5 ml 1%

Anatomy

The achilles bursa lies in the triangular space anterior to the tendon and posterior to the base of the tibia and the upper part of the calcaneus.

It is important to differentiate between tendonitis and bursitis here as both are caused by overuse. In bursitis there is usually more pain on full passive plantarflexion when the heel is pressed up against the back of the tibia, thereby squeezing the bursa. Also, palpation of the bursa is very sensitive.

Technique

- *Patient lies prone with foot held in some dorsiflexion.*

- *Identify tender area.*

- *Insert needle into bursa from the lateral aspect.*

- *Deposit solution as bolus.*

Aftercare

Avoid overuse activities for at least a week then start stretching programme. Dancers need to be careful not to over-point.

Comments

The important part of this injection is to avoid penetrating the achilles tendon and depositing the solution there. Any resistance to the needle requires immediate withdrawal and repositioning well anterior to the tendon.

ACHILLES BURSA

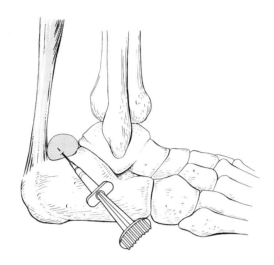

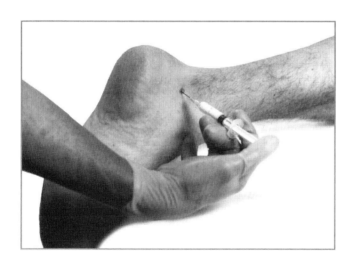

Acute or chronic tendonitis

Cause

Overuse.

Findings

Pain at lateral side of ankle or foot.
Painful: resisted eversion of the foot passive inversion.
Tender area above, behind or below the lateral malleolus.

Equipment

SYRINGE	NEEDLE	KENALOG 40	LOCAL ANAESTHETIC
1 ml	25G 5/8″ (0.5 × 16 mm)	10 mg	1 ml 2%

Anatomy

The peroneus longus and brevis run together in a synovial sheath behind the lateral malleolus. The longus then divides to pass under the arch of the foot and brevis inserts into the base of the fifth metatarsal.

The division of the two tendons is the entry point for the needle and can be found by having the patient hold the foot in strong eversion and palpating for the V-shaped fork of the tendons.

Technique

■ Patient lies supine with foot supported in some medial rotation.

■ Identify division of the two tendons.

■ Insert needle at this point, turn and slide horizontally under skin towards malleolus.

■ Deposit solution into combined tendon sheath. There should be minimal resistance and often a sausage-shaped bulge can be observed.

Aftercare

Avoidance of any overuse for about a week. Resolution of symptoms then leads to consideration of change in footwear, orthotics and strengthening of the evertors.

Comments

Occasionally the tendonitis occurs at the insertion of the peroneus brevis. The same amount of solution is then peppered into the teno-osseous junction by inserting the needle parallel to the skin to touch the base of the fifth metatarsal.

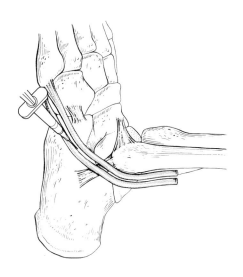

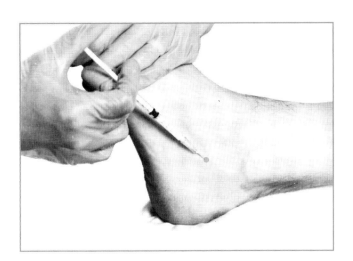

PLANTAR FASCIA

Acute fasciitis

Cause

Idiopathic, overuse, poor footwear.

Findings

Pain on medial aspect of heel on putting foot to ground in the morning.
Tender area over medial edge of calcaneus.

Equipment

SYRINGE	NEEDLE	KENALOG 40	LOCAL ANAESTHETIC
2 ml	21G 1.5–2″ (0.8 × 40–50 mm)	20 mg	1.5 ml 1%

Anatomy

The plantar fascia, or long plantar ligament, arises from the medial and lateral tubercles on the inferior surface of the calcaneum. The lesion is always found at the medial head and the area of irritation can easily be palpated by deep pressure with the thumb.

Technique

- *Patient lies prone with foot supported in dorsiflexion.*

- *Identify tender area on heel.*

- *Insert needle at 45° into the medial side of the soft part of sole of foot just distal to the heel pad. Advance towards the calcaneum until it touches bone.*

- *Pepper solution in two rows into fascia at its medial bony origin.*

Aftercare

A heel support is used for at least a week after the injection followed by intrinsic muscle exercise and stretching of the fascia. Standing on a golf ball to apply deep friction can be helpful and orthotics can be applied. Taping can also be used.

Comments

Although this would appear to be an extremely painful injection, this approach is much kinder than inserting the needle straight through the heel pad, and patients tolerate it well.

PLANTAR FASCIA

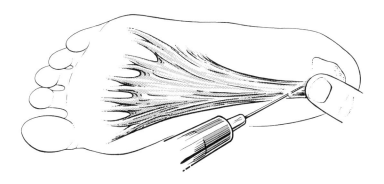

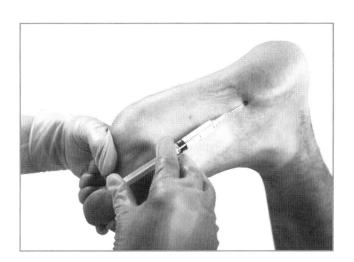

APPENDIX

PERIPHERAL JOINT & SOFT TISSUE INJECTIONS

Given in General Practice

APRIL 1991–MARCH 1996

By Dr Stephen Longworth MBChB MRCGP DM–S Med FSOM

	NUMBER OF INJECTIONS	%	
Shoulder	703	48	Upper Limb 74%
Elbow	142	10	
Wrist/Hand	234	16	
Hip	72	5	Lower Limb 26%
Knee	203	14	
Ankle/Foot	109	7	
GRAND TOTAL	**1463**	**100**	

TOP SIX INJECTIONS

Chronic Subdeltoid Bursitis	453	(31% of Total Peripheral Injections)
Shoulder Capsulitis	181	
Knee OA	150	
Tennis Elbow	92	
Trapezio metacarpal joint OA	75	
Plantar Fasciitis	70	
TOTAL ·	**1021**	**(70% of Total Peripheral Injections)**

BIBLIOGRAPHY

Assendelft WJJ, Hay EM, Adshead R and Bouter LM (1996) Corticosteroid injections for lateral epicondylitis: a systemic overview. *Br J GenPract* 46: 209–216.

Bamji AM et al (1990) What do rheumatologists do? A pilot audit study. *British Journal of Rheumatology* 29: 198–295.

Barry M and Jenner JR (1995) Pain in the neck, shoulder and arm (ABC of Rheumatology) *BMJ* 310: 183–186.

British National Formulary (Sept 1995) No 30 p. 404.

British National Formulary (Sept 1995) No 30 p. 405, 525, 402.

British National Formulary (Sept 1995) No 30 p. 522.

Cameron G (1995) Steroid arthropathy: myth or reality? *J Orth Med* 17(2): 51–55.

Casale F and Thorogood A (1985) Forum – Review of Domiciliary Consultations for Pain Relief. *Anaesthesia* 40.

Case History 1: Inadequate asepsis? (1995) *J Med Defence Union* 11(1): 11.

Clamp CGL (1994) Resources for Nursing Research: An Annotated Bibliography. *London Library Association.*

Clark JE and Lee HJ (1982) Local injections of corticosteroids. *Current Therapeutic Research.* 32(5): 761–782.

Clarke A, Allard L and Braybrooks B (1987) In: *Rehabilitation in Rheumatology – The Team Approach*, pp. 147–153. Martin Dunitz.

Clarke G (1991) Injections and NSAIDs offer the Soft Option. *Hospital Doctor.*

Cooper C and Kirwan JR (1990) The risks of local and systemic corticosteroid administration. *Baillière's Clinical Rheumatology* 4(2): 305–332.

Corrigan B and Maitland GD (1983) In: *Practical Orthopaedic Medicine.* Butterworth Heinemann p. 21.

Currey HLF and Hull S (1987) In: *Rheumatology for General Practitioners.* Oxford p. 223.

Cyriax JH and Cyriax PJ (1983) In: *Illustrated Manual of Orthopaedic Medicine.* Butterworths p. 22.

Dacre J et al (1989) Injections and physiotherapy for the painful stiff shoulder. *Annals of Rheumatic Disease.*

Dixon A and Graber J (1989) Local injection therapy in rheumatic diseases.

Doherty M, Hazleman B, Hutton CW et al (1992) In: Rheumatology Examination and Injection Techniques. WB Saunders pp. 123–127.

Dorman T and Ravin T (1991) In: *Diagnosis and Injection Techniques in Orthopaedic Medicine.* Williams and Wilkins pp. 33–34.

Drugs and Therapeutics Bulletin (1995) 33: 67–70.

Eymont MJ et al (1982) The effects on synovial permeability and synovial fluid leukocyte counts in symptomatic osteoarthritis after intra-articular corticosteroid administration. *Journal of Rheumatology* 9(2): 198–203.

Fam A (1992) Bursitis and tendonitis: a practical approach to diagnosis. *Geriatrics* March p. 25–42.

Fauno P et al (1989) A long term follow up of the effects of repeated injections for stenosing tenosynovitis. *Journal of Hand Surgery* 14(B): 242–243.

Gardner GC and Weisman MH (1990) Pyarthrosis in patient with rheumatoid arthritis; a report of 13 cases and a review of the literature from the past 40 years *Am J Med* 88: 503–511.

Garvey TA et al (1989) A prospective, randomized double-blind evaluation of trigger-point injection therapy for low-back pain. *Spine* 14(9): 962–964.

Gershon S (1983) Injecting joints and tendons with steroids. *Canadian Family Physician* 29: 2184–2188.

Geusens P and Dequeker J (1991) Locomotor side-effects of corticosteroids. *Baillière's Clinical Rheumatology* 5(1): 99–118.

Gilsanz V and Bernstein BH (1984) Joint calcification following intra-articular corticosteroid therapy. *Radiology* 151: 647–649.

Golding DN (1991) Local Corticosteroid Injections (Reports on the Rheumatic Disease - Series 2). *Practical Problems* 19: 1.

Govan ADT, Macfarlane PS and Callender R (1986) In: *Pathology Illustrated,* 2nd edn p. 865. Churchill Livingstone.

Gratter RA (1989) Arthrocentesis technique and intrasynovial therapy. *Arthritis and Allied Conditions.* D McCarty, chap 39: 647–656.

Gray RG and Gottlieb NL (1983) Intra-articular corticosteroids. *Clinical Orthopaedics and Related Research.* 177: 235–263.

Gray R and Gottlieb N (1990) Corticosteroid injections in RA: Appraisal of a neglected therapy. *The Journal of Musculoskeletal Medicine.* October: 53–70.

Gray RG, Tenenbaum J and Gottlieb NL (1981) Local corticosteroid injection therapy in rheumatic disorders. *Semin Arthritis Rheum* 10: 231–254.

Frillet B and Dequeker J (1990) Intra-articular steroid injection. A risk-benefit assessment. *Drug Safety* 5(3): 205–211.

Haslock I, Macfarlane D and Speed C (1995) Intraarticular and soft tissue injections: a survey of current practice. Br J. Rheum 34: 449–452.

Haynes RC Jr (1990) Adrenocorticotropic hormone; adrenocrotical steroids and their synthetic analogs: inhibitors of the synthesis and actions of adrenocortical hormones. In: *Godmand and Gilman's the Pharmacological Basis of Therapeutics* Godman AG, Rall TW, Niew AS et al (eds) 8th edn., *New York City: Pergamon Press* p. 1431–1469.

Henney CR et al (1993) *Handbook of Drugs in Nursing Practice.* Churchill Livingstone.

Hollander JL (1970) Intrasynovial corticosteroid therapy in arthritis. *Maryland State Med J* 19: 62–66.

Hollander JL (1985) Arthrocentesis technique and intrasynovial therapy. In: *a Arthritis and allied conditions: a textbook of rheumatology.* McCarty DJ (ed) 10th ed p. 543 Philadelphia: Lea and Fabiger.

Hollander JL, Brown EM, Jester RA et al (1951) Hydrocortisone and cortisone injected into arthritic joints; comparative effects of the use of hydrocortisone as a local anti-arthritis agent. *JAMA* 147: 1269.

Hollingwood G et al (1983) Comparison of injection techniques for shoulder pain: results of double-blind randomised study. *British Medical Journal* 287: 1339–1341.

Hopper JM and Carter SR (1993) Anaphylaxis after intra-articular injection of bupivacaine and methylprednisolone. *Brief Reports* 75(3): 505–506.

Hughes RA (1996) Septic Arthritis (Reports on the Rheumatic Diseases – Series 3) *Practical Problems* 7: 1.

Jacobs LGH, Barton MAJ and Wallace WA et al (1992) Intraarticular distension and steroids in the management of capsulitis of the shoulder. *J Orth Med* 14(2): 40–44.

Jones A and Doherty M Intra-articular corticosteroid injections are effective in knee O.A. but there are no clinical predictors of patient response. Br J Rheum (Abstract Supplement) 133: 79.

Jones A, Regan M, Ledingham J et al (1995) Importance of placement of intra-articular steroid injections. *BMJ* 307: 1329–1330.

Jubb RW (1992) Anti-rheumatic drugs and articular cartilage *Reports on the Rheumatic Disease* (series 2). *Topical Reviews* No 20.

Kendall PH (1967) Triamcinalone hexacetonide – a new corticosteroid for intra-articular therapy. *Am Phys Med* 9: 55–58.

Kennedy JC and Baxter WR (1976) The effects of local steroid injections on tendons: a biomechanical and microscopic correlative study. *The American Journal of Sports Medicine* 4(1): 11–-21.

Kerlan R and Glousman RA (1989) Injections and techniques in athletic medicine. *Clinics in Sports Medicince*, 8(3): 541–560.

Klippel JH and Dieppe PA (1995) In: *Practical Rheumatology*. Mosby p. 112.

Knight DJ, Gilbert FJ and Hutchison JD (1996) Lesson of the week: Septic arthritis in osteoarthritis hips. *BMJ* 313: 40–41.

Kraemer BA et al (1990) Stenosing flexor tenosynovitis. *South Medical Journal* 83: 806–811.

Lemont H and Hetman J (1991) Cutaneous foot depigmentation following an intra-articular steroid injection. *Journal of the American Podiatric Medical Association.* 81(11): 606–607.

Lockskin MD (1985) Corticosteroids. In *Rheumatoid Arthritis: etiology, diagnosis, management.* Utsinger PD, Zvaifler NJ, Ehrich Gem (eds). *Philadelphia; JB Lippicott* 581–599.

McCarthy GM and McCarty DJ Intrasynovial corticosteroid therapy. *Bulletin on the Rheumatic Diseases* 43(3).

McCarty DJ et al (1995) Treatment of rheumatoid joint inflammation with intrasynovial triamcinolone hexacetonide. *Journal of Rheumatology.* 22(9): 1631–1635.

Mahler F (1991) Partial and complete rupture of the achilles tendon and local corticosteroid injections. British Journal of Sports Medicine. 26(1).

Marks MR and Gunther SF (1989) Efficacy of cortisone injection in treatment of trigger fingers and thumbs. *Journal of Hand Surgery* 14(A): 722–727.

Mazanec DJ (1995) Pharmacology of corticosteroids in synovial joints. *Physical Medicine Rehabilitation Clinics of North America* 6(4): 815–821.

Moeser PJ (1991) Corticosteroid therapy for rheumatoid arthritis. Benefits and limitations. *Postgraduate medicine* 90(8): 175–182.

Murnagham GF and McIntosh D (1955) Hydrocortisone in painful shoulder – a controlled trial. *Lancet.* ii: 798–800.

Myers S (1985) Suppression of hyaluronic acid synthesis in synovial organ cultures by corticosteroid suspensions. *Arthritis and Rheumatism.* 28(11): 1275–1281.

Nelson KH et al (1995) Corticosteroid injection therapy for overuse injuries. *American Family Physician.* 52(6): 1811–1816.

Neubert C (1993) Mechanism of action and use of oral and topical non-steroidal anti-inflammatories. *New Zealand Journal of Physiotherapy.* 18–22.

Neustadt DH (1991) Local corticosteroid injection therapy in soft tissue rheumatic conditions of the hand and wrist. *Arthritis and Rheumatics.* 34(7): 923.

Noyes F et al (1977) Effects of intra-articular corticosteroids on ligament properties. *Clinical Orthopaedics and Related Research* 123.

Nuki G (1983) Non-steroidal analgesic and anti-inflammatory agents. *British Medical Journal.* 287: 39–43.

Otto N and Wehbe MA (1986) Steroid injections for tenosynovitis in the hand. *Orthopaedic Review* 15(5): 45–48.

Pelletier JP and Pelletier JM (1987) Proteoglycan degrading metalloprotease activity in human osteoarthritis cartilage and the effect of intra-articular steroid injections. *Arthritis and Rheumatism* 30(5): 541–549.

Pfenninger J (1991) Injections of joints and soft tissue: Part I: general guidelines. American Family Practice 44(4): 1196–1202.

Pfenninger J (1991) Injection of joints and soft tissue: Part II: guidelines for specific joints. *American Family Practice* 44(5): 1690–1701.

Pharmacology for Nurses (1983, 5th edition) Connechen J, Shanley E & Robson H: Nurses Aid Series, Baillière Tindall.

Physiotherapy (1990) Use of injections by physiotherapists – discussion document 218.

Principles of Medical Pharmacology (1994) Waller D & Renwick A, Baillière Tindall.

Saunders S and Longworth S (1995) Manual of Injection Therapy. *ACPOM.*

Silver T (1986) Soft-tissue lesions: injecting with confidence. *Modern Medicine.*

Simone J (1993) The principles of corticosteroid injection therapy in musculoskeletal medicine. *J Ortho Med* 15: 56–58.

Stefanich R (1986) Intraarticular corticosteroids in treatment of osteoarthritis. *Orthopaedic Review* 15(2): 27–33.

Swain RA and Kaplan B (1995) Practices and pitfalls of corticosteroid injection. *The Physician and Sports Medicine.* 23(3): 27–40.

Sweetnam R (1987) Corticosteroid arthropathy and tendon rupture. *Journal of Bone and Joint Surgery* 397–398.

Trounce JR (1990) Clinical pharmacology for nurses. *Churchill Livingstone.*

Van der Hijden GJMG, Van der Windt DAWM, Kleijnen J et al (1996) Steroid injections for shoulder disorders: a systematic review of randomized clinical trials. *B J GenPract* 46: 309–316.

Watts G and Grana WA (1983) The effects of steroids on soft tissue and intra-articular structure. A literature review. *Oklahoma State Medical Association Journal.* 76: 3–7.

Weale A and Bannister GC (1994) Who should see orthopaedic outpatients – physiotherapists or surgeons? *Annals of the Royal College of Surgeons of England* 77: 71–73.

Weisman MH (1995) Corticosteroids in the treatment of rheumatologic diseases. *Current Opinion Rheumatology* 7(3): 183–190.

Whitmore SE (1995) Delayed systemic allergic reactions to corticosteroids. *Contact Dermatitis* 32: 193–198.